ACKNOWLEDGMENTS

Just a few years ago, the idea of me sitting down to write a book was something that I would have laughed off as being a practical impossibility. The reasons for this relate firstly to my busy lifestyle and a perceived lack of time, the second reason being the issues of self-doubt and anxiety I had about putting myself out there to be scrutinised.

It truly is amazing the things you can accomplish when you commit to making something happen. I was able to overcome all the issues because, fundamentally, I believe that the contents of this book are valuable, and if it helps save or preserve just one person's sight, the journey would have been more than worth it and my measure of its success would have been met.

Of course, a journey like this so often requires the support of close people around you. So I want to thank my dear mother Charity Oguzie for her support of me and my siblings over the years. Thank you for making it easy for us to follow our own hearts and minds, while being inspirationally wise yourself. I want to thank those of you that have been sounding boards for me in the book-writing process. To all my dear friends and my godchildren, Solomon and Cyrus, I thank you for being so gracious, as I have not been around as much as I would have liked during the book-writing process. Thank you to those who read through earlier drafts of this book, your input and support was so valuable.

Finally I would like to dedicate this book to my late father Rev. Dr Bernard Oguzie; to lose you so early was difficult but I thank you for your wisdom and tough love at times. Your influence has helped me turn around my early academic failure into a career that I hope you are proud of.

Thanks and love to you all.

Know | Keeping your eyes precious

n Oguzie BSc Dip(Opt) MCOptom

Eye Know | Keeping your eyes precious

First published in 2012 by

Ecademy Press
48 St Vincent Drive, St Albans, Herts, AL1 5SJ
info@ecademy-press.com
www.ecademy-press.com

Printed and bound by Lightning Source in the UK and USA

Diagram courtesy of National Eye Institute (NEI):
www.nei.nih.gov

Illustrations: Full Collapse

Book cover: Day Three

Typeset by Charlotte Mouncey

Printed on acid-free paper from managed forests.
This book is printed on demand, so no copies will be
remaindered or pulped.

ISBN 978-1-907722-79-0

The right of Martin Oguzie to be identified as the author of
this work has been inserted in accordance with sections
77 and 78 of the Copyright Designs and Patents Act 1988.

A CIP catalogue record for this book is available from the
British Library.

This book is available online and at all good bookstores

FOREWORD

For most of us, good eyesight is something that we take largely for granted. This is not the case for everyone. The eye might be regarded as 'the window to the soul' but in more practical terms it provides the professional with a useful window to our ocular and general health.

With an increasingly ageing population the impact of sight loss or vision impairment will become more evident. Many more people will need to access eyecare services and will expect these to be available locally and provided in a convenient fashion. Access to many modern eye treatments, for example for age-related macula degeneration, are initiated by Optometrists. At the other end of the age-scale, most screening of childrens' eyes is carried out by the same professionals.

In this book, the author provides a practical and holistic approach to the role of the modern Optometrist describing the many components of the eye examination and the importance of the process.

The structure and function of the eye is described in a very readable style as are the various causes of sight problems and the various ways of allieviating them. There are many clear and well-presented illustrations in the text which help to simplify a potentially complex subject.

A section on frequently asked questions addresses many of those points that crop up regularly in clinical practice and does this with admirable simplicity.

This book will provide a useful resource to all of us who need to visit our Optometrist and provides a wealth of information for all the family.

Martin P Rubinstein PhD FCOptom FAAO

Consultant Optometrist
Department of Ophthalmology
Nottingham University Hospital

Honorary Professor
School of Life and Health Sciences
Aston University Birmingham

HOW TO USE THIS BOOK

This book focuses primarily on the work of optometrists, the optical professionals that test and examine your eyes for glasses, contact lenses and eye health problems amongst other things. For simplicity and because most people may know an optometrist as an optician, all references to optician or opticians in this book should be taken to mean optometrist or an optometrist's place of work.

The information in this book is general and may not address your own situation, so it is important to recognise that you may need to discuss specific and additional detail with your own optician. The information provided gives you a basis to have further discussions with your optician, and will hopefully help you ask questions that will get you the specific answers that you may want.

Occasional references to a diagram number e.g. Diag. 1.42 (means Chapter 1.4 Diagram number 2) may be found in a few places throughout the book. This is simply to help you understand or remember a previously explained idea or fact. Several important ideas are repeated in the different chapters for context and for the benefit of those who may not have read the previous chapters.

For explanations of tests mentioned at any point, please refer to the explanation of common tests in Chapter 1. The first chapter also contains an example sight test chart for you to look back at should you want to see where a vision reading mentioned in an example appears on the chart.

The use of scientific terms that may confuse has been deliberately kept to a minimum throughout. Explanations for one or two complex ideas are explained in ways that best help understanding, and not necessarily in the most scientifically precise way. This is designed to avoid a deeper web of complexity that may not be appropriate for this book.

All the case studies referred to are based on patients that I have cared for personally. Their names have been altered for their protection and some of the exact details of their case may have been simplified for explanation purposes.

Frequently Asked Questions (FAQs) and Tips sections are designed to address some common questions that I have been asked regularly during my professional practice over the last decade. The FAQs also serve as a great quick reference when glancing back through this book in the future.

To get the best from this book, you should read all the 'Keep Your Windows Clean' chapters, at least one of the 'Sight Through The Ages' chapters that is relevant to your age and all of the 'Make It Maximum' chapters. Of course, this book is intended to be read completely, to help you understand the changes that happen in your family's sight as well as your own.

I hope you find this book useful.

Martin Oguzie BSc Dip(Opt) MCOptom

Your feedback and comments are welcomed at:
www.martinoguzie.com or using twitter #eyeknowbook tag.

CONTENTS

INTRODUCTION

As a first year undergraduate training to become an optometrist – optician for simplification – I recall the experience of having my eyes tested by a final year student. At this point I had never had my eyes tested before, but had previously observed some aspects while on work experience. Walking into that consulting room surrounded by hi-tech instruments was surprisingly quite daunting, even for someone studying to use it all, like myself. As I took my seat on the big black chair, I was unsure of what was to come but it felt like I was about to face questioning on Mastermind.

With the test underway, I was impressed with the final year student's confidence and informative approach, telling me what she was doing as she went along. Despite her efforts, I was relieved when it was all over and couldn't help feeling like a passenger on an express train of questions and answers that left me wondering what had just happened.

As I didn't really understand why certain tests were done and whether my responses were a help or a hindrance to the process, I often felt that I was confusing the student optician. Ultimately I just brushed my questions aside, reasoning that as a first year student I was certainly not in a position to question the process, and if she didn't explain it, I didn't need to know it.

Fast-forward some 13 years later, and with a little over 10 years of experience behind me, that and other experiences along the way have influenced how I work, what I say and how I care for my patients on a daily basis. So often I hear my patients, friends and acquaintances recount unfortunate experiences at the opticians and even hospital eye departments, where they have been in and out and had no idea what just happened, were confused with jargon or were so anxious they were unsure of the usefulness of their results.

Many find the experience a passive one that they have little understanding of and therefore little control of; you just turn up, answer the questions, pay your money and trust that your best interests have been looked after.

My experience is that the optical and eye care profession is a deeply caring one, with many dedicated professionals and staff striving to get a good balance between prioritising patient care and making sure they can afford to keep the doors open. This is a balancing act I am all too familiar with, having been a practice owner myself.

I have come to realise that the eye test is a unique experience in health care, because it requires so much participation from you, the patient, that unless you understand the basic process a bit better, you can feel like that passenger on a fast-moving train heading to an unknown destination, like I did all those years ago.

Worse still is the prospect of coming back and doing it all again when your next appointment is due after a year or two 'switched off' from thinking about your eyes.

I passionately believe that through better understanding and transparency of what we do as a profession, you the patient will have a less sceptical view of the industry. Professionally, there is nothing more rewarding to an optician than the expression on a face that appreciates that their view of life has just been saved or been greatly enhanced through what we do. On the flip-side, there is nothing more heartbreaking than someone having their world plunged into darkness due to preventable blindness.

The purpose of writing this book is to help you, the reader, better understand your eyes, the eye test process and how to maintain and get the best from your sight. Having read through this book, I hope it will leave you feeling more informed and more of a participant in the care of your eyesight. The results of this might be that in between eye tests you know how to be proactive and during the eye test you feel less confused and more relaxed, leading to informative discussions between yourself and your optician.

Central to this book is the understanding that you have a part to play in the care of your eyes, but regular eye tests are essential. There is more to an eye test than buying glasses; it is essential for the health of your eyes – your most precious sense.

1. KEEP YOUR WINDOWS CLEAN

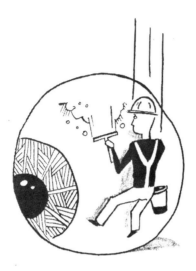

If your eyes are the window to your soul, as the popular saying goes, then your optician is the window cleaner. While they're at it, opticians also like to put their head against the glass and have a good peek at what's on the other side. A crude simplification of what your optician does, I know, but surprisingly not too far from the truth.

Let me introduce you to the two types of optician that you will come across at your local opticians. The first is the eye test optician (optometrist), trained for at least four years including a three-year degree. Their training covers everything from doing the eye and contact lens tests, including health assessment, to fitting glasses. Then there is the lesser-known, dispensing optician who will be trained for at least three years in the art of taking the prescription from your eye test and making sure your glasses are perfect.

Both jobs take much skill and patience, so both types of optician have to be registered with the General Optical Council (GOC), the body that makes sure they are up to standard for your peace of mind.

I guess that makes your optician and dispensing optician arguably the most over-qualified window cleaners you'll ever meet!

The process of 'cleaning your windows' begins with the eye test, then progresses to solving any problems found. The eye test is often a source of confusion and anxiety for many people. A process that should make seeing clearer can sometimes have the opposite result for your understanding. In this chapter I want to help you understand the basics of your eye, the eye test and some of the causes of sight problems. With the new-found clarity, I hope you will see your future eye tests in a whole new light.

1.1 KNOW YOUR WAY AROUND THE EYE

To understand even the most basic things about the eye it is useful to understand a little about the structure of the eye and the order in which the different structures are arranged. The following diagram shows the basic structure of the eye, while the notes explain some of the basic functions of the labelled parts.

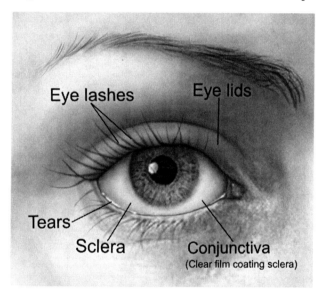

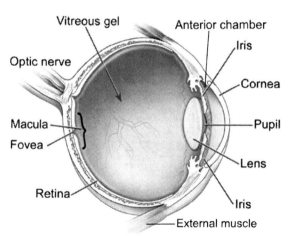

Eyelids: The soft tissue of the lids is very sensitive. It plays an important part in protection of the eye, supplying oxygen to the surface of the closed eye and tear production. Muscles in the top and lower lids control blinking.

Eyelashes: The lashes provide protection from debris falling into the eye.

Tears: The tears have three layers: oil on the outside, water in the middle and mucus on the inside touching the eye. You need all three to be balanced to have healthy tears that protect against dryness of the eyes.

Conjunctiva: This see-through film sits on top of the white sclera of the eyes and starts from the edge where the cornea meets the white. It then spreads out over the white of the eye and folds forward to cover the inside of the eyelids. It provides a protective cover to stop things falling into the eyeball socket.

Sclera: This is the tough 'white' of the eye that helps protect the internal structures, reflects light and gives the eye its rigid shape.

Cornea: The shape of the cornea mainly determines how good your far (distance) sight will be. It is not able to change shape to focus on specific objects. It must be totally transparent for optimum sight.

Anterior chamber: This is the fluid-filled space between the iris and the cornea that is regularly recycled and refreshed. The fluid helps keep the cornea healthy.

Iris and Pupil: The coloured bit of the eye is the iris. It creates and controls the pupil size by working or relaxing the muscles that are built into it. The pupil and the iris control how much light comes into the eye depending on how bright the light in your environment is.

Lens (Crystalline Lens): This lens, like a camera lens, can adjust its focus to fine-tune your sharpness. It is particularly important in helping you focus close up for reading (near) and other tasks. It must be totally transparent for optimum sight.

Vitreous gel: This transparent gel is clear and allows light to pass through to the retina while providing a pressure that holds the retina and internal layers up against the wall of the eye.

Retina: The retina is the layer made up of all the light-sensitive cells that capture the light and convert it into nerve signals to be processed by the brain, making sight possible.

Optic nerve: This is where all the nerves from the retina go out to connect with the brain. This is also where the blood vessels enter into the eye.

Macula: This area of the retina is darker in colour because there are more high resolution cells packed into this small area. It is responsible for giving you the detailed central vision needed to read text and see faces from further away. The fovea is the most central region of the macula.

Vessels: There are two main vessels that enter the eye then branch out to supply and drain the retina of blood.

Six External Muscles: Your eyes have six muscles attached to the white of each eyeball. Because the muscles are equally synchronised and balanced in strength between the two eyes, their movement is smooth and coordinated.

1.2 THE CAUSES OF SIGHT PROBLEMS

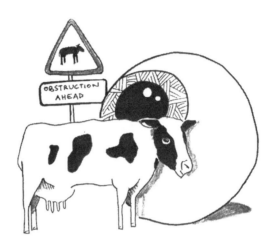

When your sight is not as good as it should be, it's a natural thing to want to know why and, more specifically, what the cause of the problem may be. There are several reasons why someone may not have great vision. These can be categorised in many ways, but for explanation purposes I will describe them in the following categories: short-sightedness, long-sightedness, astigmatism, age-related reading problems and eye disease. Later in the book I will explain the effect these may have on different age groups.

Short-sightedness (Myopia)

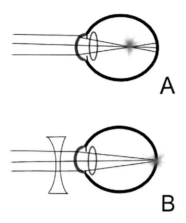

(Diag.1.21)
A) Short-sighted eye focusing light 'short' of the retina
B) correction with lenses

Short-sightedness is due to one or a combination of two things: the shape of the cornea or the length of the eyeball. For most people it is due to the cornea being more curved in shape so it bends light too much, making it focus 'short' of the retina at the back of the eye, so objects far away look blurred.

For others it can be due to having a larger eyeball than normal. This then means that while light is focused by the cornea for what might be their normal retina position, it actually focuses short because in the larger eye the retina is further back. Because eyeball size can be genetic, this type of short-sightedness is often passed down in families.

So short-sightedness affects your far sight, with things being more blurred the more short-sighted you are. People with short sight can often see well for near sight; this is because when they look at objects close up the light that was focusing short of the retina for far sight now moves backwards closer to their retina, or just past it, making seeing easier.

" **Typically, people with short-sightedness will find their far sight not so clear, while their near sight may remain clear.** "

Long-sightedness (hyperopia)

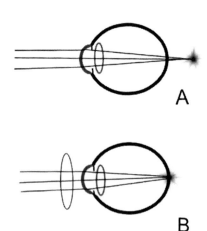

A

B

(Diag. 1.22)
A) Long-sighted eye focusing 'long' of the retina
B) correction with lenses

Long-sightedness is also due to the shape of the cornea or the length of the eyeball or a combination of the two. In most people it is mainly due to the shape of the cornea not being curved enough to bend light accurately on to the retina. A less curved cornea results in light not being bent enough and therefore focuses long, behind the retina.

Depending on how much long-sightedness you have and how well your lens is working, your far sight may still be clear because the lens in your eye can work to 'compensate' moving light focused behind the retina forward on to the retina keeping things clear far away.

When we look at objects at near sight, the light focusing at the back of our eyes moves even further behind the retina. The lens in our eyes then works to 'compensate' by moving any light focusing behind the retina on to the retina, but if you have a significant amount of long-sightedness or your lens is not 'compensating' efficiently, then things may be blurred because it is too much work for your lens to cope with.

> "**Typically, long-sighted individuals may find their far sight adequately clear while their near sight may not be so clear or comfortable.**"

Astigmatism

Astigmatism, like long- and short-sightedness, is due mainly to the curvature of the cornea. The difference here is that the cornea has two different curvatures at 90 degrees to each other. A cornea with astigmatism is often described as resembling a rugby ball on the surface, while a cornea without astigmatism is described as resembling a football.

The main problem with astigmatism is that it causes more complex distortions of the image you see. It requires correction of both curvatures separately in the affected cornea so that the image is sharp and distortion-free.

Age-related reading problems (presbyopia)

The lens in the eye has a relatively limited life of useful focusing. So most people find that they start to notice the early signs of sight problems with reading from about 40 years of age and onwards. The exception may be moderately short-sighted people, who continue to read well at a comfortably close distance without any reading glasses beyond this age.

The lens is an oval disk-shaped structure with an outer layer shell. Throughout life this outer layer of the lens constantly replaces old cells with new ones and when it does this, the old cells get pushed towards the centre of the lens. By the time we get to 40 years of age, it is starting to get really packed out with these old cells, resulting in the lens being harder and less flexible. As this progresses, you will find that reading becomes more of a problem and you will need to use reading glasses more as time goes on. The lens eventually becomes so packed that it doesn't have any flexibility to focus for you at all.

Eye disease

A disease causes cells to function abnormally, leading to a range of problems from minor body changes requiring no treatment to potentially life-threatening conditions. As with the rest of the body, the eye can be affected by many diseases directly or can be affected indirectly by diseases in other parts of the body. These conditions range from conditions you are born with to conditions you are more likely to get with age, gender, race, family history and so on.

While many diseases can damage the sight, it is often true that the earlier detection takes place and treatment starts, the better the prospect that sight can be protected from permanent or further damage. It is also important to remember that many conditions will creep up on you without warning; the first sign you get may be when it has caused permanent damage to your sight or eye. It is essential to remember that, for this reason, the benefits of regular sight tests cannot be replaced by the information in this or any other book.

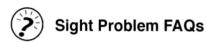 **Sight Problem FAQs**

1. Will my sight improve with regular wear of my new glasses?

In adults, the development of the eye is complete. That is to say that all the cells of the retina and other visual structures are at the maximum maturity and have stopped developing. Glasses and any other sight-corrective device or procedure simply redirect the focusing of light on to the retina, so that the light-sensitive cells can use it and help you see well.

There is no conclusive evidence that wearing your glasses regularly results in your sight being any better or worse without glasses over time. For it to do this, the glasses would either have to change the shape of the front surface of your eye, the cornea, or change the performance of the cells of the retina at the back of the eye. There is no evidence that it can do any of these things in the adult eye.

However, children under the age of seven to eight years have eyes that are still developing. As a result, if your child is told to wear glasses regularly by your optician, this can give the cells of your child's eyes the clarity they need to stimulate better development and better resolution. So in the case of young children with eyes that are still developing, the answer to this question could be yes if worn as advised.

2. I have family history of eye problems, will it affect me?

Having a family history doesn't mean that you are definitely going to be affected in exactly the same way as your relative, if at all. How likely you are to be affected depends on factors such as what the condition is, whether it is your parent, a sibling or a more distant relative. Having a family history of a condition that can be passed down can pose a risk for you or your children, but thankfully it's not guaranteed.

Your optician is trained to be aware of the implications of your family history of eye problems, that's why they ask and may do extra tests to investigate and explore your eye health. Family history is always an important thing for your optician to consider when testing your eyes. So be sure to know if you have any relevant family history of conditions such as diabetes, glaucoma, heart or stroke problems.

Less common conditions such as retinitis pigmentosa, corneal dystrophies or unknown causes of blindness that you may be aware of are all relevant things to mention too.

3. What happens if the optician finds a serious problem with my eyes?

Occasionally an eye test will lead to the discovery of problems of concern requiring further investigation or treatment. In these situations, your optician will refer you to a specialist eye doctor for investigation, treatment or an opinion. This can be done directly to the eye hospital or through your own doctor. Your optician will usually suggest the urgency of attention needed for the referral based on how serious the condition is to your sight. The other option that your optician has is to manage and monitor non-serious conditions for change over time.

 ## Sight Problem Tips

If you have never had a sight test before, then you cannot be sure that there are no problems going on inside the eye, even if your sight appears great. The eyes are so good at adapting and 'making do' with a gradual reduction of sight that you may never know until things become too blurred. Blurred vision may be correctable with glasses but sometimes correction is not possible for different reasons.

An example would be the situation of the adult with an eye that has not developed normally because their childhood eye problem was not referred to an optician before it was too late.

Here is an interesting trick to test whether your sight is as good as it should be. Clench your fist to create a pinhole through your fingers. Make sure the pinhole you create is as small as possible while still letting a clear beam of light through. Look through the pinhole with one eye only and focus on something written in the distance. Compare that with your vision in the same eye without looking through your fist. You can swap eyes and try it with the other eye. Does your sight look sharper through the pinhole?

How it works: central beams of light coming through your pupils do not need focusing at the back of the eye, but all the other light coming through that is not central does. So if you need glasses, your eye doesn't focus these non-central beams sharply so things look blurred and they hide the clarity from the central beams too.

When you look through a pinhole you are cutting out the non-central beams leaving just the central beam which focuses sharply at the back of the eye. This is why screwing your eyes up helps you see better and why seeing in bright light is better than in low light, because your pupils get smaller in bright light and larger in low light.

As interesting as this test is, never take it to mean that you shouldn't get your eyes tested properly by an optician.

1.3 UNDERSTANDING THE EYE TEST

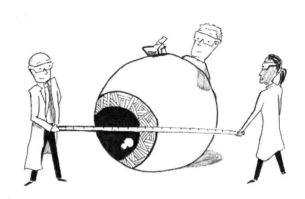

The aim of the eye test

When you have your eyes tested, your optician wants to get accurate information from you and make accurate observations about your eyes with the simplest tests that are possible. The results of the test can be used to make a decision about whether your sight needs correction or not and whether referral to hospital is needed. The other important information we get from your eye test is to do with how healthy your eyes are. Usually at the end of the test the results are discussed with you and your options are explained.

The eye test, which is referred to by some as the sight test or eye examination, can be thought of in three parts: Part 1 - History and symptoms, Part 2 - Your responses and Part 3 - Our observations.

" **...your optician wants to get accurate information from you and make accurate observations about your eyes with the simplest tests that are possible.** "

Part 1 History and symptoms: This is your opportunity to explain what problems you are having and what medical or family history of eye problems you may have. The more information you give about the questions asked, the more helpful this will be to your optician. I recall a case of a patient of mine who refused to tell me what was wrong with her, insisting that it was up to me to find out and tell her. Unfortunately it doesn't work like that, I explained.

What you tell your optician may lead to them doing more tests for investigative purposes that wouldn't have been done otherwise. It is also useful to make sure you mention whether you use computers much and about what position the screen is, and any hobbies or interests for which you rely on good vision. It all adds to getting a clearer picture of what your visual habits and needs are, which is important when thinking about what correction options to recommend to you.

Part 2 Your responses: This is where many people get really stressed out. The most common fear with this part is that you are giving the wrong responses, confusing the optician and your glasses or contact lenses will be incorrect. Well, relax because it is not often that this happens and when it does your optician will usually know.

Remember that if it appears difficult to make a decision about whether things look better in option '1 or 2' as you may be asked, that will usually be because it is difficult to tell. I often put my patients at ease by telling them that as we get near the point of their best vision it becomes difficult to see differences; a bit like splitting hairs, it's hard to be precise. So just say what you think and if you can't tell between the options, say so. It's OK, your optician will know what's going on.

Part 3 Our observations: This part of the test often gets people unnecessarily worried because it involves checking the health of the eye. The tests done here may require bright lights to be shone at your eyes, puffs of air or drops going into the eye. Be reassured that the eye test usually involves no pain and, more often than not, patients are pleasantly surprised to find that any fears they had about the tests were unnecessary.

Common Tests used

Tests are done in Parts 2 and 3 of the eye test and can be done in any order depending on who is doing it. Different opticians may develop their own slightly different ways of doing things. Your optician has many different tests that they can choose to do, depending on your symptoms, problems, age or risk factors you may have. We will now look at some of the more common tests done and what they are for.

Part 2 tests

Sight Test Chart

A	6/60
BC	6/36
DEF	6/24
G H I J	6/18
KLMNO	6/12
P Q R S T U	6/10
V W Q Y Z A B	6/9
C D E F G H I J	6/7.5
K L M N O P Q R	6/6 (20/20 American)
S T U V W Q Y Z	6/5

(Dig. 1.31) Example of test chart arrangement

There are a few types available, but traditionally they are arranged like the one in the image shown here. Your optician will ask you to read the letters on here and some of the other tests will be done on this chart too. Many opticians now have computerised test charts which offer a lot more flexibility.

Reading vision is tested on a handheld chart that you will be given. Average vision is the 6/6 line on the chart, which is the same as 20/20 vision in America. Borderline vision for safe driving is considered to be at least the 6/9 line, but lower down the chart is preferred.

Testing the coordination of your eyes

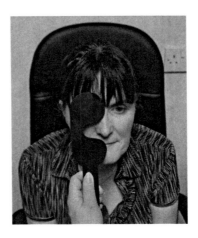

This is the 'cover test' and involves covering each eye, one at a time, as in the image shown. The test requires you to look at a target far away while the person testing you covers your eyes one at a time. It is often done with a target at close reading distance too. The purpose of the test is to check that the eyes are coordinated and do not have a tendency to turn in any direction, often causing images you are looking at to split into two (double vision).

Testing the movement of your eyes

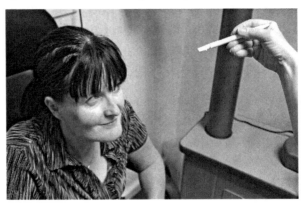

The 'motility test' is done either with a penlight or some other device that you can follow. The test requires you to keep your head still and follow the light as it is moved in front of you. This test indicates whether you have full and normal movement of your eyes. If you don't, this test can indicate which of the six muscles in the problem eye may be at fault.

Testing how well your eyes turn in

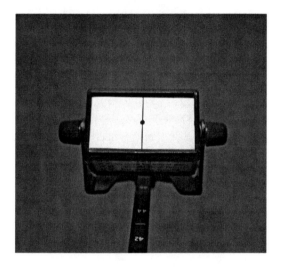

The 'NPC (Near Point of Convergence) test' is often done with the special ruler with a spot and line on a chart attached to the ruler as shown. The chart can be moved forwards and backwards along the ruler when testing. The test requires you to watch the spot and line, while the ruler's cheek rest is placed on your cheeks. You must then indicate when the line splits into two as it is moved down the ruler towards your nose. This test indicates if you are likely to have problems converging (turning in) your eyes to look at things close to you, such as with reading or computer use. This test can be done in other ways without the ruler.

Testing how well your eyes focus

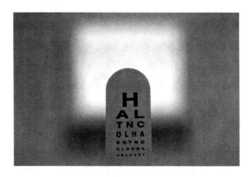

The 'amplitude of accommodation test' is used to check how well your eyes focus close up on an object. This is usually done with a few lines of text on a special ruler or with a reading chart. The test requires you to read the text as it is moved closer towards your nose and indicate when it starts to go blurred. This test indicates how much focusing ability your eyes have remaining.

Testing how well your eyes are aligned

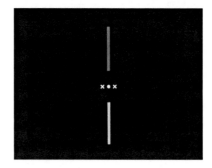

The 'fixation disparity' test can use an OXO or the XOX arrangement of the test, shown above. This test is done with special filter lenses on, and requires you to watch the central O and indicate if either of the bars moves out of centre and towards the Xs. This test mainly indicates whether your eyes are out of alignment or not, giving clues to the nature of any sight problems you may have.

Testing how relaxed your focus is

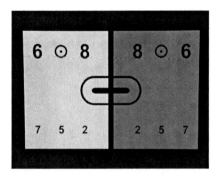

The 'duo chrome test' involves looking at the black-coloured rings or figures, depending on the chart, and indicating whether they appear clearer on the red or green background. The test indicates how relaxed your focus is. When your focus is relaxed with the correct lenses in place you should see the black rings on the red and green as close to equal as possible, although this may not always be achievable.

Test for astigmatism

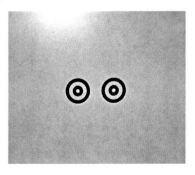

The 'cross cylinder test' is done as part of the check for the strength of your glasses and is done with a special lens called a cross cylinder, held on a stick. You will be asked to look at a target, usually some rings, spots or a circular letter. The lenses are flipped in two positions and you will be asked to choose which appears clearest and most circular. This test indicates whether you have football (no astigmatism) or rugby ball shaped eyes (astigmatism) and helps find the strength of lenses needed to make things look clearest. Astigmatism is a common reason why people need glasses.

Part 3 tests

Pupil Reactions

This test is done with a bright light source that is shone into each eye one at a time. How your pupils react to this light can indicate whether there is damage to the back of the eye affecting the flow of nerve signal up through the eye to the brain.

Detailed looking at the front of the eye

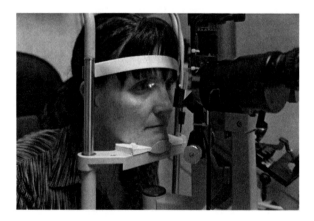

The device shown is a 'slit lamp.' Although it has several uses, its main function is a microscope for looking at the surface of the eye in detail. You will be required to put your chin on the chin rest and forehead on the forehead rest before the examination starts. Other devices can be attached to it such as a device to measure the pressure in your eyes, as they do in many eye hospitals.

The pressure test

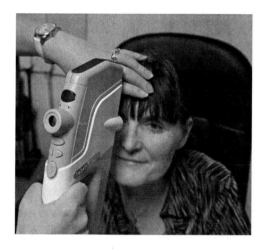

The device shown is the most common way of doing this test in optical practices, although there are other ways. The device blows a puff of air on to your eye as you watch the light inside the device and tells your optician if the pressure inside your eye ball is normal or not. It is one of the tests for glaucoma. Glaucoma can be explained in simple terms to be when the pressure in your eye becomes too high, causing a risk to your sight.

" It is important to remain anxiety free when having your sight tested. "

Looking at the back of your eyes

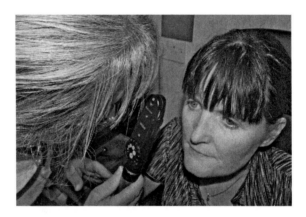

This device, known as an 'ophthalmoscope', is used to have a look through your pupils and into the back of your eyes to check that everything is healthy. You will be asked to move your eyes in different positions to allow a thorough look into your eyes. Whilst it is a common way of looking at the back of your eyes, there are other methods as well. Some opticians may get you to sit at the slit lamp while they hold a small lens in front of your eye to get a magnified view of the back of the eye. This may be done instead of or as well as using the ophthalmoscope.

Finding your glasses prescription

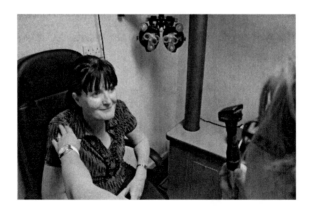

A device called a 'retinoscope' is used to identify whether you are short-sighted or long-sighted and by what strength. You are simply required to look towards the target, usually the red and green lights on the chart. Light from the device is then shone towards your eyes while lenses are placed over your eyes.

Testing for blind spots

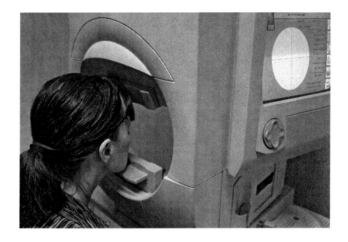

The 'visual field' machine comes in a variety of shapes and sizes. It tests whether you have any blind spots in your field of vision. Blind spots may be caused by damage to the back of your eye or along the pathway from your eye to your brain. The test involves looking into the machine with your head and chin on the rests.

When the test starts, one eye will be covered at a time, you will be asked to watch a coloured light straight ahead all the time, while looking out for any white spots of lights that may flash up in the corners of your sight. When you see a white spot, you respond by pressing a button, or in some machines you tell the person testing you how many spots you see.

Photography

Photographic equipment is becoming more widely available; it offers the advantage of being able to save the image of the back of your eye for comparison at future visits. This means that any problems can be accurately monitored for slight changes or, if a new problem develops, we can look back to confirm that it was not present before. You are required to place your forehead and chin on the rest and watch the target as directed. Several photographs will then be taken.

Drugs used occasionally during the eye test

Drugs are sometimes used as part of the eye test, and are used by your optician to help them make a decision about what they can or cannot see. The drugs are all eye drops and are in very low doses. Here are the common drugs that your optician may use from time to time.

Dilation drops - These drops are used to make your pupils bigger so that your optician can have a better look through to the back of your eye to investigate. This is normally used when someone complains of certain suspicious symptoms or if visibility to the back of the eye is difficult – for example, due to small pupils or cataract. These drops may make things appear more blurred until the effect wears off in about three to six hours.

The main issue you may experience with these drops will be increased sensitivity to bright lights due to your pupils being large outside in the light when normally they would reduce in size to prevent dazzle. This can be resolved by wearing sunglasses until the effect of the drops wears off. Driving is not advised when these drops have been used because it may affect how safely you will be able to drive.

Relax focus - These drops hold your focusing fixed so that a more reliable prescription for glasses can be achieved. It is most commonly used for young children who may not be very cooperative when it comes to keeping their eyes on a target object when they are being tested. Without the drops their focus wanders, making the test result unreliable. These drops will sting for a few seconds before settling down. They will leave the vision blurred until they wear off which may take between six and 24 hours.

Anaesthetic - These drops serve to numb the sensation of pain and touch on the surface of the eye so that the eye can be touched without excessive discomfort. It is commonly used if the eye pressure is being measured using the contact technique, which involves touching the eye with a special probe. The effects will last for about 15 minutes but it is important to remember not to rub the eye if you can help it until the effects wear off, just in case you unknowingly scratch your eye.

Dye (Fluorescein) - This dye is orange in colour and as long as not too much is put in, it shouldn't be too obvious in your eye out in the daylight. It is used to assess the quality of your tears – for example when trying to diagnose dry eye. It is also commonly used to investigate any damage to the surface of the eye of contact lens wearers or anyone that might have objects unexpectedly entered into the eye.

Any areas of damage on the surface of the eye will absorb the orange dye and, using a special blue light on the microscope, these areas of damage stand out for your optician to examine. Without the dye it can be impossible to see the areas of damage because things will otherwise look normal.

Eye Test FAQs

1. *How often should I have my eyes tested?*

    This varies from individual to individual, but as a guide anyone aged 70 and over should be seen every year; those aged 16 years and over who don't have any health problems should be seen every two years; children aged six and over every year; and those below the age of six need to be seen every six months at the most.

    These guidelines are general and may be more or less frequent depending on what your optician thinks is appropriate for you. Never feel that you have to wait to bring your child in if they are having any significant sight problems; you can always contact your optician and check whether the symptoms require earlier eye testing.

2. *How do I know if I am giving the optician the right answers so that my glasses are prescribed correctly?*

    This is probably one of the biggest sources of anxiety for many having their eyes tested. I would reassure you that while they are not looking for specific responses from you, your optician is well aware of whether or not the responses you are giving are helping to get the best sight from your glasses. If your optician becomes aware that your responses are being affected by your anxiety or inability to see a difference, they will know what to do, that's part of their expertise.

It isn't often that anyone confuses their optician, although it may seem to you that you may be contradicting in your responses. In fact, the reason it can be very difficult to make a decision in the eye test is usually because, as we get nearer to your optimum prescription strength, it becomes harder to tell a difference between the options presented – a bit like splitting hairs, difficult.

3. *What can my optician tell from looking into my eyes and what do they see?*

Many people have no idea that when your optician looks into your eye they can see all the blood vessels, the retina and other features at the back of the eye. This is how we are able to tell so much about your general health. Medical conditions that affect your blood vessels, such as diabetes, hypertension and arteriosclerosis, can affect the vessels in the eye, allowing your optician to get an indication of your health. There is a wide range of information that can be obtained from looking at the back of the eye.

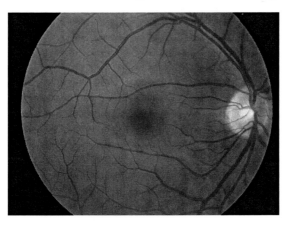

(1.32) The normal view inside the eye.

Eye Test Tips

It is important to remain anxiety free when having your sight tested. This will make you feel more at ease and will help make you feel more confident about your responses in the test. It is helpful to be honest with your optician if you are anxious or worried, by explaining how you feel at the start. This gives them the opportunity to reassure you and go at a pace that suits you.

Once you are in the chair, take a few slow deep breaths in and out to help relax yourself. Then just respond honestly to the questions; if you are not sure of anything, say so or ask for things to be repeated for you if it helps. The key is to avoid guessing, unless your optician specifically tells you to guess.

1.4 WEARING GLASSES

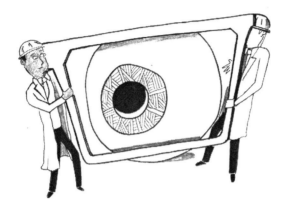

In my experience, one of the biggest barriers to feeling more in control of the whole experience of having your eyes tested at an optical practice is the confusion surrounding glasses and the range of products, coatings and treatments available for your lenses. Being able to understand the basics will help you control the cost of your eyewear by buying what you want and knowing why you want it. You will be able to ask the best questions to get what you want and you may also consider buying new products you wouldn't have chosen before.

Choosing your glasses after the eye test is a very important part of the test. There is no point having a great eye test only to get poor advice outside of the test room resulting in you spending a lot of money on glasses that you can't see with. Mistakes happen and that is a normal part of working with precise optical measurements, but a registered dispensing optician supervising or dealing with the purchase of your glasses can help reduce these mistakes through their expertise.

Understand your glasses prescription

If you have ever had your eyes tested and received your copy of the prescription, only to be totally confused about what all the numbers mean, you are not alone. It is not an easy thing to explain and attempts can often cause more confusion. It can be useful to have a basic understanding so that, for example, you can see for yourself how your prescription strength is changing from visit to visit. You are entitled to a copy of your prescription after your eye test with any optical practice.

Your prescription can be taken anywhere and informs the optical company how to make the lenses that will give you the best vision, as found by your optician. The most important, but confusing, part of the prescription information is the table containing numbers arranged similarly to those in the example below.

	SPH	CYL	AXIS	DVA	ADD	NVA
R	-2.50	-1.25	90	6/6	+2.00	N5
L	+5.00	-2.50	45	6/5	+2.00	N5

The prescription details are split into R, for right eye details and L, for left eye details. The table then has columns for SPH, CYL, AXIS and ADD. Sometimes there may also be a column for VA. What follows is an explanation of what the different elements of a basic prescription mean.

SPH is short for sphere. The number in here may have the positive (+) or negative (-) sign before it. This number is the main part of the prescription: correcting long-sightedness with a positive power number or short-sightedness with a negative power number. The smallest number you will usually see here is 0.25 because we usually change lens powers by 0.25 (or quarter) steps.

So in the above example, this individual is short-sighted in the right eye by 2.50 diopters (diopters is the unit of lens power). However they are long-sighted by 5.00 diopters in the left eye.

CYL is short for cylinder. The sign before the number here is normally determined by the way your optician chooses to write it. The vast majority of opticians make this number a negative sign in their issued prescription. The CYL and the AXIS both relate to correcting astigmatism – the condition where the surface of the eye has two different curvatures 90 degrees to each other.

So instead of being spherical like a football, the surface of the eye is more rugby ball in shape. The SPH is the lens power needed to correct the main curve, while the CYL is the lens power needed to correct the other curve of the rugby ball shaped eye's surface.

AXIS is a measurement in degrees. You can think of it as instructions telling the optical lab what direction to place the CYL power in your glasses, to correct the curved surface that is causing the rugby ball shaped (astigmatism) eye. When it is lined up correctly, things appear sharper and without distortion.

VA stands for visual acuity. This is simply the vision you are getting on the chart when you have the lenses on. Not all prescriptions will have this section; if it does, it may ask for far sight readings, near sight readings or both, as in our example.

How we record vision:

Distance - As standard, most test rooms use a chart with letter sizes equivalent to being six metres away. So when we record visual acuity (vision) we write it as a fraction (one number over another) with the 6 on top, to represent that the distance the letters are being viewed from is six metres or equivalent.

The bottom number changes depending on the size of the letters you can see. The smaller the bottom number, the better your vision. Average vision also has a bottom number of 6, making the VA value 6/6 – the same as 20:20 vision, the American equivalent. In our example we can see that for far sight this individual has average vision in the right eye, but better than average vision in the left eye because he has VA of 6/5 in the left eye.

Near - This is usually recorded with a number after the letter N, and again, the smaller the number the better the vision. N6 may be considered average, but most people should be able to see to N5 if they have average vision in their far sight, like our subject in the example.

ADD is the reading addition strength. The ADD is the additional strength needed on top of the far sight strength for tasks such as reading and knitting. The number in the box is usually the same for each eye and the number must be added to the SPH part of the main far sight prescription to give you the actual reading glasses prescription. Using our previous example, we get the following results for the separate reading and computer glasses.

Reading	SPH	CYL	AXIS	
R	-0.50	-1.25	90	
L	+7.00	-2.50	45	

Your actual prescription may be written a little differently from the example we have looked at here but that doesn't mean it is wrong. With the above information, hopefully you now have a basis to ask for specific clarification from your optician or dispensing optician without being totally confused.

Lens materials

So now you understand your prescription better, it's time to discuss your options when having your glasses made up. The first consideration will be what lens material to go for. The options are glass or plastic and, in reality, almost all the lenses sold today are plastic. Glass lenses used to be the most popular choice due to their great optical quality and toughness. However, advancements in plastic lens and coating technology mean that most lenses sold today are plastic rather than glass.

The main advantages of plastic lenses compared to glass are weight and safety considerations. Plastic lenses are lighter than glass making them easier to live with daily because there will be less weight on your face and less pressure for your glasses to slide down your nose. Plastic lenses will not shatter in the same way as glass when broken so are safer if an accident occurs.

Plastic lenses can be standard resin or polycarbonate in material. Polycarbonate is a very tough plastic, so tough in fact that it is used in bulletproofing and safety eyewear because it is so impact-resistant. Polycarbonate also has good optical quality and 100% UV protection. However, it has two flaws: its soft surface can be prone to scratching, but can be treated with a hard coating, and it is sensitive to acetone-based solvents which can weaken and damage it, so these should not be used.

High index lenses

The refractive index (index for short) of a lens material tells you how dense the material is, and therefore indicates how thin the lens may appear compared with another material. The more dense a material, the less of it you need to achieve the desired power so the lenses can be made thinner.

So when you are offered thinner lenses at the opticians, it is worth finding out the index of the material compared to your current lenses or standard plastic lenses. Standard plastic lenses would have a low refractive index of 1.49 while lens materials with the highest refractive index would be 1.74 or a little over, giving the thinnest lens edges.

Lens types

Some of the options you will be faced with when making a decision on new glasses will include whether to have separate glasses for far sight and near sight or whether to have multifocal lenses, which combine both far and near sight into one lens. We will now look at the options and what they mean.

SVD Single vision for distant sight. These lenses are made to correct your far and general sight only and not the near sight. They are normally for driving, walking, watching TV and so on.

Advantage: Consistent far sight, large seeing area for driving and other tasks. Easy to get used to.

Disadvantage: You may not be able to read close up with them. You may have to keep swapping between these and other glasses.

SVN Single vision for near sight. These lenses are made to correct your near sight specifically and so you may find everything blurred beyond arm's length. They are normally prescribed for reading, knitting and so on.

Advantage: Consistent sight and large reading area for reading books for long periods of time.

Disadvantage: You can't look up and see across the room. You may have to keep swapping between these and other glasses.

SVI Single vision for intermediate sight. These are made to correct your sight for middle distances and are ideally for looking at computer screens, reading music on a stand and so on.

Advantage: Consistent sight and a large reading area for computer use.

Disadvantage: You can't look up and see across the room. You may have to keep swapping between these and other glasses.

Bifocals. These are made combining a reading area in the distant sight lens. The shape of the segment area can be made to different shapes depending on your needs. Bifocals have a clear line separating the distant from the near sight lenses.

Advantage: They are relatively straightforward to get used to, providing good consistent sight. They are also convenient, putting distant and near glasses into one pair. This means you no longer need to change between two pairs of glasses or carry two cases around with you.

Disadvantage: Going up and down stairs can be an initial problem for some as well as reflections off the line on certain bifocal designs. They are not the best option if you are going to wear them when using the computer, unless they are customised for that purpose. The reason for this is that the reading area on the lens is so low down that you will have to hold your chin up constantly and get closer to the screen to keep things clear. This will inevitably result in discomfort and tension due to bad posture.

Trifocals. These are made combining distant, intermediate and near sight lenses all into one lens. Trifocals have a line separating all three sections.

Advantages: You tend to get wider vision for computers and reading than you would with a basic varifocal. Steady sight and no need to swap between these and other glasses.

Disadvantage: The lines of the segments may annoy some people and cosmetically they may not be to everyone's liking.

Varifocals. The lens combines distant, intermediate and reading sight into one lens. The difference between it and a trifocal is that a varifocal has no visible lines running through it.

Advantage: looks good cosmetically, has distance, intermediate and reading in one and they are very convenient. No need to keep swapping between these and other glasses.

Disadvantage: The sides of the lens are usually out of focus so you have to turn your head more. The reading and intermediate area may not be as wide for computer use as some people would like.

Varifocals also tend to cost a little more than single vision lenses. The increased head movements required may take some getting used to.

Remember that there is no right or wrong decision, just what is right for your needs at work, home or any other environment in which you will be using your glasses. Many people get put off by multifocal glasses due to fears over how they will adapt to them, but the reality is that only a small proportion of people can't get on with them.

Varifocals usually come with a guarantee that allows you to change the lens to something else if you can't tolerate them. Most optical practices are very helpful in this regard, so ask about this and any other concerns you may have.

Lens add-ons

There are several different optional add-ons that you could have on your lenses to enhance their performance in different situations. Here are some of them explained.

Anti-reflection (or anti-glare) coating - The purpose of this add-on is to cut down light reflected off the lens surface. Up to 16% of light may not make it to your eye when wearing glasses because it is reflected away. This can make things look less sharp, introducing more fuzziness round lights, particularly when driving or reading in low light. The coating can reduce the reflections to just 2%, making things appear clearer with better contrast. This is also good if you have a known problem with glare.

Scratch-resistant coating. This does exactly what it says: it makes plastic lenses more resistant to scratches. It does not promise to make them scratchproof, so beware.

UV coating. This coating does a more thorough job of blocking out harmful ultraviolet radiation from getting through to the eye. Although plastic lenses do quite a good job of blocking UV anyway, the benefits of protecting our eyes further cannot be overstated due to the potentially harmful effect on the back of the eye and contribution to cataract development.

Tint treatment. Tints are great because of the different colours they are available in and their shade providing benefit in the sun. They should be accompanied by a UV coating, because the eye behind the tinted lens will have a larger pupil than without it, which means that UV radiation can have easier access to the back of the eye. Polarised lenses are also tinted, to at least 50% level. Polarised lenses are particularly known for being great at reducing glare.

Photochromic lens treatment. These lenses change with the light, going dark outdoors and staying light indoors. The reaction in the lens has improved greatly over the years and they serve as a very convenient solution for light-sensitive individuals and anyone who wants tinted lenses for everyday use. They rely on UV light to work, so if you are in a car with all your windows up, they may not work so well because the car windows may absorb all or most of the UV light.

Hydrophobic coating. This coating is designed to resist grease and oily substances on the surface of the lens making them easy to clean. It also makes the lenses more resistant to water collecting on the lenses when they would normally steam up.

"Convenience is the main aim of multifocal glasses, not constant wear..."

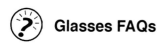 **Glasses FAQs**

1. Will my eyes get dependent on glasses if I start wearing them regularly?

This is a common worry of many that stops them wearing their glasses as often as they should. The reality is that if your glasses make a big difference to your sight, then wearing them regularly is likely to make you feel that you need them more.

However, the reason for this is not that the glasses are making any physical changes to your eye or the muscles of the eye. It is more due to the fact that your visual system is very good at 'making do' with what you can see, so when your vision is blurred long enough you will get used to the sight and feel it is adequate.

New glasses that make things a lot clearer can make your visual system aware and get used to what it has been missing, so it then becomes hard for your brain to go back to the blur you were used to. Strangely enough though, if you managed to go without your glasses for some time your visual system will again learn to 'make do' with the blurred sight without your glasses. So do not worry about wearing your glasses regularly if you are advised to by your optician.

2. Do multifocal glasses have to be worn all the time?

Many people wrongly assume that the point of multifocal glasses is that they should be worn all day, every day, or regularly in every case. This is not necessarily the way that multifocal glasses have to be worn by everyone. The benefit of multifocal lenses such as varifocals is that when you do have them on, you have everything you need in one pair of glasses. Because far, near and middle sight are all built into a varifocal lens, you won't need to carry two or three pairs of glasses around with you, swapping between them often.

Even if you do not wear glasses for far sight, a multifocal can still be useful to stop you putting reading glasses on and taking them off as you constantly change focus from reading or computing to looking across a room. Convenience is the main aim of multifocal glasses, not constant wear, although you can choose to wear them constantly if your optician advises that you can.

3. *Why does the anti-glare coating on my lenses make them attract fingerprints, can I have this and other lens add-ons removed from the lens later?*

Anti-reflection coatings, or anti-glare as they are sometimes known, are very effective at dealing with the wasted light reflecting off the surface of your lenses. They are so effective that the grime and fingerprints that used to be hidden by the reflections now become obvious to see. So in reality the coating doesn't create more fingerprints, but it does make them more visible as a result of doing its job so well.

So the best way to avoid getting fingerprints on the lens is simply to avoid touching the lens, and using lens cleaning sprays periodically. Many anti-reflection coated lenses now also come with hydrophobic coatings that resist grease and grime from fingerprints, making them easier to wipe away.

With the exception of a standard tint, once lens add-on treatments are applied, they cannot usually be removed later without damaging the lens. Standard tinted lenses can sometimes be made lighter in colour afterwards but usually only if they do not already have other surface treatments applied to them.

 ## Glasses Tips

- A registered dispensing optician is an expert on everything to do with glasses. Do not mistake them for a well-qualified optical assistant who is trained 'in-house'. If your practice employs one, don't be afraid to ask them all your product-related questions.

- When choosing the frames for your glasses remember that the best quality frames tend to last longer with careful use. So while they may cost more, they could quite easily last twice as long as a budget pair. This means that in future you can reuse the frames and have new lenses put into them should you wish. So if you hate choosing frames and would rather stick with what you are comfortable with for as long as you can, this is worth remembering when choosing.

- If, on the other hand, you are someone who likes to change looks regularly, you may still want your frames to last as long as possible so that you can reuse the frame and keep it in your collection for different occasions.

1.5 WEARING CONTACT LENSES

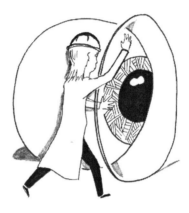

Contact lenses are a great way to correct your sight as an alternative to glasses. They offer many advantages to the user and they come in many different lens types to suit many situations. Over the years, the cost of lenses has also come down to reasonably low prices; now they are a viable alternative to glasses for many people, although back-up glasses will still be advisable in case of emergencies.

The advantages of contact lenses include the fact that they do not steam up, they are safer for sports, some can correct far and near sight together, they are available as coloured prescription lenses and so on.

Lens Types

Hard contact lenses (rigid gas permeable lenses). Also known as RGP lenses, these hard lenses are less commonly fitted in practice now, mainly due to them being very uncomfortable initially until your eyes get used to them. Their advantages are that they are considered healthier for your eyes than soft lenses. Because they're small in diameter they still give the surface of the eye, the cornea, space to breathe naturally, unlike soft contact lenses which cover the entire cornea.

They tend to be very good at correcting vision, often resulting in better vision for wearers of complex prescription glasses compared to soft lenses. These lenses are also very long-lasting, with one lens having up to two years' recommended maximum use before replacement.

Soft contact lenses. These are the main contact lenses being fitted today, due to their instant comfort, convenience, appeal for sport and variety of lenses available.

We will focus our attention now on the soft lens types that exist on the market and what they do.

1. Daily disposable contact lenses. These lenses are worn for one day only and thrown away at the end of the day.

The benefits of these contact lenses include the following:

- Good comfort due to being very thin and having high water content. Once on the eye they are often instantly comfortable, making them easy to get used to.

- Convenient because they do not require any cleaning. This makes them great for busy people or those with concerns about maintaining regular care of their contact lenses.

- The idea of having a fresh lens in the eye daily is something that attracts many to daily disposable lenses.

Disadvantages of daily disposable contact lenses include the following:

- Regular wear may prove a little more expensive than having lenses that are reused more than once.

- Drying out of the lenses can often be an issue for some people, depending on the brand of the lenses and the activities they're involved in, as well as the environment they are in at the time. Prolonged computer use and hot environments tend to be the most problematic for some.

Contact lens manufacturers are constantly improving their lenses, and newer daily disposable lenses tend to be improved upon the limitations of those available previously.

2. *Reusable contact lenses.* These lenses are reused and replaced monthly or two-weekly, typically depending on the brand of the lenses. These are probably the most common type of lenses in use today.

The key advantages of these lenses include the following:

- Often represent best value in price for regular wearers.

- Available in the widest range of strengths and fittings to suit most eyes.

- Good comfort and tend to be more resistant to drying out than daily disposable lenses.

The disadvantages of reusable contact lenses include the following:

- Require regular cleaning and care.

- You have to make them last longer.

- By the end of a month's reuse, they may not feel as good as a fresh pair.

3. *Multifocal contact lenses.* These lenses correct far and near sight in one. Unlike bifocal or varifocal glasses, you do not need to move your head or look through a particular part of the lens. So in theory they should provide effortless far and near sight. In practice, these lenses tend to work with varying success on different people depending on their prescription strength for glasses and the size of their pupils.

Advantages of multifocal lenses are as follows:

- Conveniently improves near and far sight in one lens.

- Available in daily disposable lenses, reusable and continuous wear lenses that you sleep in.

The disadvantages of multifocal contact lenses include the following:

- Comfort is a little worse than non-multifocal contact lenses because they are thicker.

- They do not work for everyone due to limited reading power availability and the individual's pupil size and prescription.

Other methods of dealing with far and near sight: When multifocal contact lenses do not work there are two other options that can be explored by your optician, the first of which is a technique called mono-vision. Mono-vision involves correcting one eye with a contact lens for far sight and adjusting the other eye for near sight. As strange as it sounds, when a good balance in lens power is reachable between the two eyes we find that you will experience good far and near sight, without eye strain. Mono-vision is particularly good for occasional or social use. The other option is to correct far sight fully in both eyes and wear simple reading lenses over the contact lenses when you need to see near objects and text.

4. *Continuous wear lenses (Sleep in)*. These lenses are made from a special silicon hydrogel material rather than the normal hydrogel types used to make standard contact lenses. This makes them so breathable that you can sleep in them for a maximum of 30 days continuously before removal. However, unless you have a really good reason to wear them for that long, I always advise removing and cleaning the lenses weekly to minimise any hygiene risks.

Advantages of continuous wear contact lenses include the following:

- Almost completely breathable, allowing oxygen to pass through to your eye very easily.

- They are more resistant to drying out of the lens than standard lenses.

- Can also be worn like reusable lenses and removed daily for maximum health benefits, but allowing all-day wear.

- This more breathable material is also available in some daily disposable lenses too.

Disadvantages of continuous wear contact lenses include the following:

- Can be an excuse for laziness with the care of the eyes and lenses.

- Are more rigid than standard lenses, so may not be as instantly comfortable.

- Increased risk of contact lens-related eye problems when worn continuously for up to 30 days.

"Don't let the thought of touching your eyes put you off, you will soon get used to it."

Contact Lens FAQs

1. *Can my child wear contact lenses?*

Many children dislike the idea of wearing glasses regularly, although this is less common with all the great children's ranges of fashionable glasses frames available today. Nevertheless, a significant number will ask for contact lenses as an alternative to glasses.

Strictly speaking, there is no age limit to contact lens wear, but due to growing eyes and the fact that kids get themselves into all sorts of situations and environments which could make hygiene of the lenses difficult, caution is advised when fitting children or young people with contact lenses.

Most opticians would be reluctant to fit children under the age of 16 years with contact lenses for regular wear unless there is a very good reason. If you have a child with a moderate to high prescription who wants contact lenses for occasional wear for sports or social use, then this could be a possibility depending on the child and whether they have your support as their parent.

There could be other situations where your optician would fit a child with contact lenses, but it is down to their discretion. Wanting them because the child doesn't like glasses is not a good enough reason, because they will still need glasses as a back-up to contact lenses, and keep in mind that the ongoing cost of contact lenses may be significantly higher.

2. Can I sleep in contact lenses and what will happen if I do?

It is important that you follow the advice given to you by your contact lens optician. Not all lenses are the same, and the guidelines for lenses are there for good reasons. There are only a small number of lenses that you can sleep in, the rest are to be worn for no more than 12 hours maximum in a day unless your optician tells you otherwise.

The main danger of lens over-wear, or sleeping in lenses when you shouldn't, is that you start to deny your eyes oxygen. A lack of oxygen can cause the eye to get creative, resulting in vessels starting to grow into the cornea from the white of the eye in an attempt to try and supply the cornea with oxygen. The cornea doesn't normally have vessels in it because it needs to remain clear, so this can potentially cause you sight problems due to glare from scattered light hitting these vessels if a significant number form in the cornea.

Infections or red painful eyes are other consequences of over-wear, while a future intolerance to contact lenses may also result if you make it a regular habit. If you need or want to sleep in contact lenses, see your optician to get fitted with the correct lenses.

3. I want contact lenses but I don't know if I will be able to get the lenses in and out, how will I know?

Rest assured that you are not the only one that has felt this way, in fact most current wearers of contact lenses felt the same before getting started! I compare learning to put contact lenses in and taking them out to learning to ride a bike: tricky to start with but once you learn you'll wonder why you struggled in the first place. The key is patience and having a teacher who is patient and observant. Don't let the thought of touching your eyes put you off, you will soon get used to it. Essentially, the only way you will know if you can do it is to give it a go.

 ## Contact Lens Tips

Contact lens wearers often suffer dryness of the lens or eye when using them for work on computers or driving for significant periods of time. This is often due to the type of lens you wear, the environment and your blinking efficiency. Lenses with a high water content, such as daily disposable contact lenses, are most prone to drying out, while the materials in silicon hydrogel lenses, such as the lenses you can sleep in, are less affected by drying out.

Blinking tends to be a problem because when we do any task requiring concentration for a significant amount of time, such as computer use or driving, we all stare more and blink less. When we do blink, it is often half-blinks leaving a central area of the eye or contact lens that has not been wet properly. This leads to water evaporating more from the contact lens because it is not being rewet properly by blinking, leading to dryness.

When using computers or driving while wearing contact lenses, be aware of your blinking, taking care to blink regularly and fully so that your tears get spread over the whole lens surface. Avoid long periods where a fan or heater is blowing directly in your face and make sure the environment is not too hot; these can all make drying out of the contact lens more likely.

1.6 LASER SIGHT CORRECTION

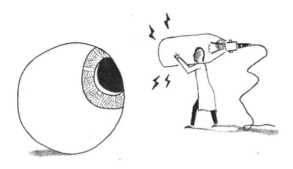

Laser treatment is one way of correcting your sight that interests many people. In the early days of the technology there were significant limitations with the procedure in that it was only available to people with certain prescriptions. There were also more problems associated with the procedures due to the newness of the technology, so the risk of undesired complications was higher.

Now the technology has advanced significantly with superior lasers and techniques that have dramatically improved the results achieved for patients' sight. However, the biggest drawback for many is the fact that laser correction still doesn't correct both far and near sight in each eye at the same time. This means that if you are a short-sighted individual in your 40s who needs glasses for far sight, but can read a book fine at near sight without glasses, then laser surgery may correct your far sight but leave you needing glasses for near sight reading from the age of 40 years and onwards.

For many people in their 40s, it defeats the object of laser correction if they still have to wear glasses at all, while for others this is not a problem as long as they can get up in the morning and not have to reach for their glasses as their first action to allow them to get around the house. In an attempt to solve this problem, the laser industry offers some people the option of correcting one eye for far sight and the other for near sight, in a technique similar to mono-vision as carried out for some contact lens wearers.

It sounds like a strange arrangement, but if the power difference between the two eyes is balanced just right it can provide a comfortable solution because the visual system makes enough sense of the image from each eye without them being too incompatible. So with contact lenses it can be shown to work well but whether you want it as a permanent change made to your cornea is another matter, due to the slight compromise you may experience to your 3D vision and depth perception.

Everyone is different so a discussion with your surgery provider about what would suit your circumstance is advised and will inevitably take place. Surgeons are increasingly offering people non-laser alternatives to correct both far and near sight all in one with cataract-style operations, where your lens is removed and replaced with an artificial varifocal-type lens (combines far and near sight power in one lens).This may prove to be the new trend in sight corrective surgery in the years to come.

" **...the technology has advanced significantly with superior lasers and techniques that have dramatically improved the results achieved for their patients...** "

Laser correction is offered using several techniques and laser options depending on your prescription or circumstance. Your laser correction provider will have a more detailed discussion with you about the options. Here is a brief overview of the two main laser techniques you may be offered currently.

LASEK (Laser-Assisted-Epithelial-Keratomileusis)

The procedure involves the following:

- Anaesthetic eye drops are applied to the eye to remove the sensation of the surgery on the eye. The eyelids are held open with special clips to prevent blinking.

- A flap is created by making the cornea more supple using alcohol on the surface before simply crumpling the top layer (called the epithelium) to the side creating a flap.

- The flap created is folded back and a computer-controlled laser then zaps the exposed layer of the cornea very precisely to reshape it to give you the best vision. The laser and computer is so precise that it can even track when your eye moves off focus and still laser in the exact location. This only takes a minute or two.

- The corneal flap is folded to fit exactly back in the right place. The whole process takes less than 20 minutes.

After the treatment you will usually be given a special contact lens to wear to help the healing process for a few days. You may also be given some eye drops to use for a few days, but you will be able to see straight away and within a few days the vision should be significantly clearer.

LASIK (Laser-Assisted-In-Situ-Keratomileusis)

The procedure involves the following:

- Anaesthetic eye drops are applied to the eye to remove the sensation of the surgery on the eye. The eyelids are held open with special clips to prevent blinking.

- A flap is created by shaving a precise layer off the cornea using a special precision surgical device with a sharp blade.

- The flap created with a hinge is folded back and a computer-controlled laser then zaps the exposed layer of the cornea very precisely to reshape it to give you the best vision. The laser and computer is so precise that it can even track when your eye moves off focus and still laser in the exact location. This only takes a few minutes.

- The corneal flap is then replaced to fit exactly back in the right place. The whole process takes up to 20 minutes.

After the treatment you will usually be given some eye drops to use for a few days, but you will be able to see straight away and within 24 hours the vision should be significantly clearer.

The main difference between the two procedures is that LASEK creates a flap closer to the surface of the eye and LASIK goes deeper. LASEK may carry an increased risk of post-operative glare problems and longer recovery time, but you may still be eligible for it if you have a thinner cornea. LASIK, on the other hand, is probably the most common technique in use now for its accuracy and ability to produce the best visual results, but it does require you to have a cornea of a certain thickness.

Two significant laser advancements that have really improved the clarity of vision achieved while minimising complications are IntraLase (femtosecond laser) and Wavefront technologies. These may be mentioned to you in the early stages of your consultation. Both technologies can be applied to LASIK and LASEK, but tend to be offered as options by some laser correction providers.

IntraLase is a super-precise laser that can be used to create the flap on the cornea instead of using a blade, as in LASIK, or just crumpling the top layer to the side to create the fold in LASEK. The use of the special laser in the IntraLase process means a very accurate flap can be created, making healing quicker and complete, without risk of micro-scars.

Wavefront laser technology is used during the reshaping process to allow super-customised reshaping of the cornea. This is particularly useful if your cornea has irregular thickness. This is not corrected as precisely with non-Wavefront lasers, or with glasses for that matter. As a result, Wavefront has the potential to give you slightly better sight than you might expect from glasses. Tests and measurements done before your operation will highlight if you are likely to benefit from Wavefront for better definition to your sight.

If you are going to have laser sight correction it is worth ensuring that IntraLase and Wavefront are part of your procedure to ensure the best chance of an outcome that exceeds your expectations.

Advantages of laser correction:

• Prospect of being glasses-free for under 40-year-olds.

• Relatively simple and quick procedure.

• No weight of glasses on the nose.

- Mono-vision offers the possibility of being glasses-free for over-40s.

Disadvantages of laser correction:

- Can't be used to correct near and far sight at the same time in each eye.

- Mono-vision may affect 3D vision and depth perception slightly.

- Can be viewed as expensive.

- Not everyone is suitable.

Laser Correction FAQs

1. *Would you recommend laser correction?*

The decision to have laser sight correction is one that you have to arrive at yourself. I wouldn't put anyone off having it unless there was good reason to. It is important to do a little research yourself to make sure you are comfortable with the risks associated with surgery of this type.

Many if not all the leading laser sight correction companies offer free or low-cost initial consultations, so take advantage of it to ask your questions and satisfy yourself that your expectations are realistic. If everything sounds fine and you are happy with the clinic and surgeon, then I would be happy that you have made a good and informed decision.

2. *Am I suitable for laser correction?*

The question of suitability comes down to several considerations which won't be known until you have some suitability tests at the laser clinic. To work out if you are suitable the clinic will take several measurements of your eyes, such as the thickness of your cornea, the curvature of your cornea, the length of your eye using ultrasound and so on.

They will also want to know about your eye and general health. Your glasses prescription will also be important; many clinics ask that you prove that your prescription has not changed for at least a year, if not longer. If it has changed, it may continue to do so straight after your surgery.

3. Does the effect of surgery wear off?

The benefits of the surgery will be undone if your glasses prescription starts to change again. So it is in your best interest to have surgery when there is evidence from looking at your last two sight test prescriptions that things have not changed much. This will help you avoid disappointment.

If you had a significant prescription for glasses before surgery, then it is unlikely to deteriorate to that level again. I have seen many patients who after 10 years still remain glasses-free even with the earlier laser sight corrective techniques.

 Laser Correction Tips

Shattered expectations are often the cause of dissatisfaction with laser correction. To make sure your expectations are realistic and that you are totally at ease with the decision you are about to make, you may want to do some research and visit up to three different clinics before making your decision. Many of the clinics offer free initial assessments to check your suitability and discuss the options with you.

You will also have the opportunity to ask questions to satisfy yourself of anything you are not sure about. The benefit of visiting different clinics is to make sure you are happy with the information you are receiving about which technique is best for you and the cost. Most surgeons will happily answer your questions and let you know the results of previous patients they have treated with prescriptions similar to yours.

2. SIGHT THROUGH THE AGES

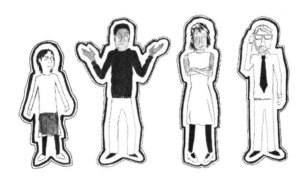

A decade of testing sight and examining eyes of all sorts of people of every age and background throws up many observations. Here I have condensed some of my observations into four significant age categories and the visual hallmarks that I have found to be clearly present in the average person within this age category.

These four groups are: children, the age in which rapid change can happen; the 20s-30s, the age when change may be more stable, resulting in complacency; the 40s-50s, the age when sudden near sight problems causes increased awareness; and the 60s+ when the effect of age causes degenerating sight.

Throughout the ages there are different visual trends and changes to sight that may be more specific to an age group. We also tend to find that some conditions are more common within certain age groups, although not exclusive to that age group. Regardless of age, there will always be the need to be vigilant about your sight and even more so about maintaining the health of your sight through regular visits to your optician.

2.1 THE AGE OF CHANGE: CHILDREN

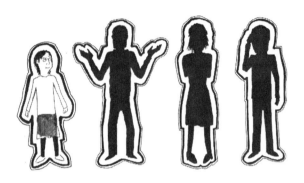

The importance of regular sight tests

If ever there was an age group most at risk of suffering a long future of poor sight, it would be children up to the age of about seven to eight years. Beyond this age there may be less of a risk, but continued rapid growth means that they may be more at risk of rapidly changing sight until their growth slows down beyond the age of 16 years. It is for all these reasons that children must have their sight tested and eyes examined on a regular basis.

So why is the age limit of seven to eight years thought to be a significant cut-off, you may be wondering? Well, the reason is due to this age limit being traditionally understood to be the cut-off of the 'plastic period' of eye development. The plastic period is the period in which the retina and its nerve links are still developing, and can be influenced by external things affecting how clearly light forms an image at the back of the eye.

After the plastic period, things become 'set' and not thought to be any longer influenced by external factors. The worry for the child that has a significant prescription for glasses which is not detected and corrected before the plastic period is that the retina's cells never develop good resolution once development becomes set.

In order for the cells of the retina to develop maximum resolution, they need to have sharply-focused light on them. The eye test will check that this is happening normally or whether your child needs glasses to help make this happen.

Age-related changes

Children's sight can change significantly and quickly as they grow and become teenagers, as I have already said. The following case gives an example of the nature of the change that may be typical of the way things can progress quickly with normal growth in some children.

Sam is a 15-year-old lad who came to see me. He has a long history with us, dating back to the age of four years. When he started coming to us he was typical of many young children, in as far as he had slight long-sightedness of about +1.00 in each eye and vision that was a little worse than good adult vision of 6/6 equivalent (see Diag. 1.31), although only simple tests with pictures were possible at this age.

Sam's mother reported no noticeable problems with him. Looking back, we see that as Sam starts school and grows we examine him every six months until the age of six years. The observation from his test results are that Sam's sight is improving and by the age of five years he is seeing to good adult levels of vision and his long-sightedness is reducing, being now zero in the right eye and just +0.25 in the left eye.

By age six Sam returns, reporting that he has started to notice slight problems with seeing the board at school, but books are clear to read. The test results show that Sam has now developed short-sightedness of -0.50 in the right eye and -0.75 in the left eye, making his vision noticeably more blurred for far sight. Now that Sam is old enough to have a more thorough eye test, it is also discovered that he may have a mild colour vision defect.

He is prescribed his first glasses and we continue to see him every six months instead of the usual yearly visit for the over six-year-olds, so his changing prescription can be monitored. As he is monitored over the years, he is confirmed as having a mild colour vision defect, good coordination and movement of his eyes, but his short-sightedness continues to get worse quickly.

Aged 11, Sam has short-sightedness of about -1.25 in the right eye and -1.75 in the left eye with some astigmatism too. His sight without glasses is now quite blurred looking at far objects, but great when reading at near distances. At the point of me testing this young boy, aged 15, he has deteriorated short-sightedness of -1.50 with slight astigmatism in the right eye and -2.25 with slight astigmatism in the left eye. Glasses correct his vision on the chart down to the very good level of 6/5 in each eye.

Sam's case highlights several issues about the changes that may result in the sight as children develop and grow. Sam's parents were wise to bring him in for his first sight test at age four, an important period for any child as they start school and many new learning experiences. Their development here onwards will be greatly influenced by how well they see, so even if they don't appear to have any sight problems, children should have their eyes tested.

If your child is experiencing any sight problems, it may be a sign of something requiring treatment of some sort, so please seek advice from your doctor or optician. In the normal development of their eyes, it is typical to find that children may be slightly long-sighted. As children grow we tend to find that their long-sightedness reduces, hopefully stabilising around the zero prescription mark when most of the child's growth stops.

Long-sightedness may need correcting if it is severe or causing strained eyes, but in Sam's case it was deemed small enough to not need any correction. If you look back to the earlier explanation of long-sightedness in this book, you will understand that the young eye deals very well with long-sightedness compared to short-sightedness.

The process of reducing long-sightedness doesn't always happen as described, and the danger is that in some children this process can be very fast and overshoot the zero prescription and develop into short-sightedness instead. The worry here is that the far sight will quickly become blurred for the child. As we see in Sam's case, his eyes continued into short-sightedness, and will probably carry on beyond 15 years old, but hopefully will stop once he stops growing. Children below the age of six years will need to be tested at more regular intervals of about six months or less because they are still in that critical plastic period where their sight can be influenced and improved with the appropriate treatment.

"Computers and prolonged reading can cause certain known discomfort issues..."

Visual trends amongst the young and their possible problems

It doesn't seem too long ago that personal computing was the preserve of the affluent and the business community. Technological advancements and lower prices now mean we have personal computers in most homes and mobile phones within the reach of most people. The fastest take-up of all this technology is undoubtedly children, who are all frantically connecting with each other around the world.

I come across many parents who are concerned about the amount of time their children spend looking at computer and mobile phone screens. If you're concerned about your children, firstly I want to reassure you that there is currently no definitive evidence that reading, computing and watching screens for extended periods of time causes permanent damage to the eyes, or leads to a particular eye condition for that matter.

However, given the developing nature of young eyes and the fact that no conclusive evidence doesn't mean anything is definitely safe, I would advise caution. Computers and prolonged reading can cause certain known discomfort issues, so the usual advice of regular breaks should apply for young people over shorter periods of time.

So as a guide, teenagers should probably take a 10-15 minute break to get up and move after one hour with regular pauses in between the hour to relax their focus by looking across the room and blink more. I would advise that children aged seven years and younger should be allowed to play and use computer devices as part of normal learning, but it would probably be wise to avoid excessive unsupervised use.

Five common childhood problems

1. *Squint.* This is the situation where a child develops an eye that turns out of alignment. It is often due to a child below the age of seven to eight years having a large amount prescription for glasses that goes undetected and uncorrected. It is also common to find that the prescription for glasses is bigger in the eye that turns compared to the other eye. The lens in the affected eye constantly wants to work harder than the other eye, trying to keep things in focus, which leads to pressure for the eyes to turn.

   Over time this pressure causes an imbalance in the muscles that turn the eye, resulting in a squint. Long-sightedness tends to cause eyes that turn in, while short-sightedness tends to cause eyes that turn out. You can also have squints that turn up, down or rotate in or out. Another cause of squints could be weakness in one of the six muscles responsible for turning each eye, causing an imbalance.

   Disease process or nerve damage can also be less common causes of squints. In any case, urgent assessment is needed to establish the cause and whether treatment is possible. Treatment depends on cause and can vary from prescribing glasses, muscle exercises, surgery or no treatment at all.

2. *Colour vision defect.* Often inaccurately described as colour 'blind', colour vision defects are actually quite common and can be passed down in the family. Red-green defects are the most common colour vision problem but are rare in girls, with only about 0.5% of females having a problem compared with 8% of males having a problem. Sam, the young boy in the case discussed, had a colour vision defect which was detected early on and his parents were advised.

This is important to identify at school age because if the school is made aware of the nature of the defect it may influence the colours their teachers use in helping to educate children. I usually reconfirm colour vision status at future visits for young children when their understanding of the tasks is better, as I did with Sam. Reassurance is given to parents that, while it will always be there, your child will lead a perfectly normal lifestyle. They will just need to be aware that they may be restricted from certain careers where normal colour vision is essential.

3. *Lazy eye (Amblyopia).* This is when a child develops an eye that does not see as well as the other eye even when corrected with glasses. It can often be present in an eye that has a squint (turns out of alignment) too. The reduced vision is due to the child below the age of seven to eight years not being given corrective glasses early enough, so a blurred image has been falling on to the retina cells at the back of the eye.

The retina cells then fail to develop the connections with the brain that would make high resolution images possible. Treatment has to be in the 'plastic period' below the age of seven to eight years to give the best chance of reconnecting the connections. During this 'plastic period' the cells of the retina are still trying to improve and fine-tune their connections; once they stop trying, improvements are not possible.

Treatment for lazy eye is patching therapy, a process where the good eye is patched up, forcing the so-called 'lazy' eye to do its best to see. It then responds by trying to fix and fine-tune its connections with the brain, improving the sight. The older the child, the less likely it is to work.

4. *Need for glasses.* Significant prescriptions for glasses require correction from as early an age as possible. Some parents worry that their optician has mentioned that there is a minor prescription, but has not recommended glasses for their child. The reasons should be communicated to you clearly; if they are not, then be sure to ask.

As a guide: very small amounts of short-sightedness and astigmatism are likely to need glasses, while small amounts of long-sightedness may not need glasses. However, every case is different, so your optician will treat your child as an individual and make a professional judgment about what is best for them.

5. *Eye diseases.* Fortunately they are not too common in practice but, like with adults, childhood eye diseases can vary widely and many can be as a result of things going on in other parts of the body or inherited conditions in the family. Many will not be obvious to the child, so examination of the back of their eye, which is part of every eye test, is important in detecting any problems.

Children's Sight FAQs

1. What tests will be done?

Just simple tests to get an idea that the child's sight is progressing normally, and to look out for any problems with coordination of the eyes and any other developmental issues. Their far and near sight will be tested, along with the coordination and movement of their eyes. Further tests may include checking for colour vision and 3D vision problems. Other more advanced or adult tests, such as measuring the pressure inside the eyes, are not normally carried out on children.

Sometimes your child may need to have drops put into their eyes to help relax their focus. This is so that a more reliable prescription can be obtained even if their eyes wander around the room.

2. How do you test children's vision if they don't read?

Vision is usually measured using different sized pictures or by asking your child to match similar shaped letters on a handheld card to the ones on a far sight chart. These kinds of tests simply rely on your child being able to recognise differences between letters and shapes, which is usually within the capability of many preschool children.

3. Why do children's prescriptions change so fast?

Essentially the answer to this is down to their rapid growth towards adulthood. It is normal for young children to be slightly long-sighted without it causing them a problem that needs correcting with glasses.

As they grow, this long-sightedness reduces itself in a process with the technical name of emmetropisation as the child grows. It is to be hoped that by the time they stop growing things will remain stable at close to zero prescription. During the period of growth, therefore, rapid changes are not unusual in some children.

 ## Children's Sight Tips

Because of the playful nature of kids or the gradual way some problems develop, some parents miss signs of their children having sight problems. Key telltale signs of sight problems to look for in children include the following:

1. Closing one eye - A child that tends to close one eye may be experiencing double vision. This double vision is not present with one eye closed, so your child may close one eye trying to make the sight less confusing.

2. Getting nearer to objects in the far sight like the white board or the TV - This may indicate a problem with your child's far sight, needing correction. It can sometimes just be a habit that they have picked up, but it needs checking.

3. A child with a white pupil - This can sometimes be seen in photographs in the same way you may have a red eye image, or you may observe a whiteness in colour through the pupils. This may be one of the most common (but still rare) childhood tumours of the eye, retinoblastoma, which needs urgent action.

These observations need checking urgently by your optician. However, do not hesitate to contact your optician if you observe any of the more common sight and eye problems or get the feeling that things aren't right.

2.2 THE AGE OF COMPLACENCY: 20s-30s

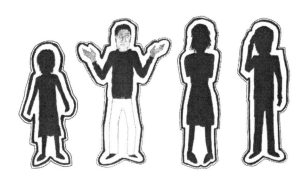

The importance of regular sight tests

This is a period in life when the eyes are in their prime and less associated with eye or sight problems. The very fact that many people will feel very comfortable with their eyes and sight at this period of life often reinforces a sense of complacency about the care of their eyes. Taking their eyes for granted is perhaps a result of how well they do their job when everything is working well.

So why are eye tests essential at this period of life, you may ask? Well, if children's vision represents a period of frequent change, then the 20s-30s represents a period of more subtle change. The danger with subtle change is that the visual system is wired to pay more attention to rapidly changing levels of sight. As a result, you may never be aware of reduced vision until it reduces to disabling levels, and then it may be too late to restore it.

This is an all too common occurrence up and down the nation's optical consulting rooms, and something I have witnessed many times. On the whole, the cause of the reduced vision in these individuals is optical and can be corrected with glasses, contact lenses or laser correction. Occasionally it can be due to eye disease, requiring referral for hospital investigation or treatment.

Safety on the roads while driving is an important consideration when it comes to looking after your eyes. Gradual deterioration of your sight can put you in the situation where your sight becomes dangerously low and you may never know. Most people are under the impression that if their sight deteriorated significantly they would know, which is a reasonable assumption to make, but this is often not the case. The following case highlights this and the whole complacency issue that arises when you naturally get comfortable with your sight and take seeing for granted.

Monica is a 24-year-old IT professional who came in for her first eye test. She drives daily and uses computers a lot as the main part of her working day. She informs me that her sight is great for driving but she has started experiencing tired aching eyes at the end of the working day and occasional mild headaches. Having completed the eye test, Monica was surprised by the results.

It turns out that her far sight was not as good as she had thought it to be. Her right eye was only able to see to 6/9 line on the chart and 6/15 with her left eye. The sight test showed that she was short-sighted in both eyes, but had worse sight in the left eye. Her prescription for glasses was found to be -0.50 in the right eye and -1.50 in the left eye with a small amount of astigmatism in this eye too. For near sight she was seeing well with both eyes.

Monica described her sight as being great for driving when, in reality, it was likely to be very borderline for safe driving, particularly in low light situations. This demonstrates the problem arising from your eyes adapting to gradual deterioration, allowing us to make do with lower quality vision.

When corrected with glasses, Monica was able to see down to the 6/5 line on the test chart with either eye, which represents better than average sight. The implications for her driving with borderline or unsafe sight include invalidating her motor insurance and the risk of harming others or being harmed on the road.

Monica also mentioned tired aching eyes at the end of the working day. The results of testing her sight and examining the health of her eyes revealed that this problem is likely to be due to a combination of dry eye and having a significant difference between the prescriptions in her eyes. Dry eye can be due to medical problems such as arthritis, certain medications or blockage of the ducts that release liquids making up the tears.

However, none of these applied to Monica, so the dryness of her eyes was put down to her working and driving habits, as well as environmental. She will often drive for an hour with the air conditioning blowing in her face; she then gets to work and sits in front of her computer for hours at a time.

Whenever we engage in any task that requires us to concentrate, such as driving and computer use, and stare for significant lengths of time, our blinking frequency reduces and often they become half-blinks instead of full blinks. This then leads to drying out of the eyes due to exposure making the eyes feel more sore, tired and sensitive. You may also get more dilated blood vessels on the white of the eye, making the eyes look slightly red.

The difference in Monica's prescription strengths between the two eyes may contribute to her problems when working on the computer for long spells of time, due to the fact that the eye may require different focusing. This difference in focusing power required by the two eyes can result in conflict between them, leading to eye strain. Eye strain is sometimes described as a pulling sensation in and around the eyes which can, in some instances, lead to a headache around the forehead.

Age-related changes

The age of complacency, as I describe it, is a period in life when many of us enjoy a period of peak performance from our eyes and sight. By the time they reach 20 years of age, most people would have undergone the fastest and most dramatic change in growth that they are likely to experience in life. At the same time, their sight would have completed its development below the age of 10 years and is now stabilising from the effects of growth.

So between the age of 20 to the late 30s you may well enjoy great and stable sight that makes you feel that everything is, and will always be, perfect. On the other hand, you may be in the smaller but significant group of people who may still experience rapid and dramatic change through their 20s and 30s. Change in this case may be linked to family history of large amounts of long-or short-sightedness due to a larger or smaller eyeball size than normal.

How your sight and prescription changes in your 20s and late 30s is not all that predictable, so it's hard to know when or where your prescription strength for glasses is likely to stop if it hasn't already done so in your 20s. As uncomfortable as it is to know, there's not a lot you can do. Keeping up to date with your eye tests is important; your optician will rule out medical causes for any rapid change to your sight, such as thinning of the cornea or fluid build-up in the cornea or macula.

In your 20s-30s there is little, if any, effect of ageing on the eye, so for the most part it is definitely a time in life to enjoy great sight if you have it. Resist the temptation to become complacent because things can go wrong or change at an unpredictable time and often with a pace that creeps up on you unknowingly.

Visual trends amongst the group and their possible problems

As well as regular computer use for work and increasing social use, there is a big uptake of contact lenses and, increasingly, laser correction amongst this group. The visual trend amongst the 20s-30s is driven by the desire to be free from wearing glasses.

For many wearers, the desire to be free from glasses starts in their 20s, if not before. As soon as they're able to, more people in this age group than any other are motivated to try contact lenses for social, sporting and regular wear. For many, the natural progression from contact lens wear is laser correction, a trend in development within this generation and perhaps predominantly amongst those in their late 20s and early 30s.

"For many wearers, the desire to be free from glasses starts in their 20s, if not before."

The increasing popularity of laser correction has been driven by the marketing, the obvious appeal and the huge advancements in laser and computer technology that have made the procedures available to more people with a wider range of prescriptions. As a result, many of the problems with early laser correction techniques have been minimised.

Naturally, as with any surgery, there is still the risk of complications. These complications can range from dry eye, glare or less sharpness than you had with your glasses. These are all issues that need to be thoroughly investigated and understood before you embark on treatment. Laser sight correction is an expanding industry but I would expect that in the years to come, it will still be mainly individuals in their 20s-30s that will choose to have laser correction.

So does this pose a threat to opticians and their livelihood, you may wonder? Well, not in my view because you will still need to maintain regular eye tests for monitoring the health of your eyes. I also believe that many laser patients in their 40s will still choose reading glasses to improve their near sight, a problem that laser surgery does not solve.

Five common conditions affecting this age group

Many of the conditions here can also occur at any age, but within the 20 to 30 age group they are just some of the conditions that may be frequently seen by opticians. As part of the regular eye test, the symptoms you report will help your optician identify what it is that is wrong with you and what course of action is needed to help you.

1. *Conjunctivitis and infections* - Conjunctivitis is the inflammation of the transparent skin which covers the white of the eye. Inflammation of any tissue tends to cause

redness, swelling, discomfort, discharge and pain. The redness is due to blood vessels becoming larger, making them more visible. Conjunctivitis is often due to bacterial infection, requiring only antibiotic eye drops.

The danger is that some inflammatory conditions such as iritis can be a lot more aggressive, needing referral for more serious medical treatment. The consequences of these can be both sight- and, very rarely, life-threatening if left untreated. Your optician will need to ask you some questions about the symptoms you are getting and will examine your eye in detail.

2. *Headaches* - Are a very common reason for many people coming to get their eyes tested. It is also a very good reason to have your eyes tested because headaches have many potential causes and your optician can help to rule out some of the most dangerous ones. The causes of headaches can be sight-related or non-sight-related.

Sight-related reasons can include eye strain associated with needing glasses, eye coordination and movement problems, and so on. Non-sight-related causes can be migraines, high blood pressure or, less commonly, sinister things like tumours or aneurisms. As well as testing for sight-related reasons, your optician can test your field of vision, which can help rule out anything more sinister going on in the head. Consult your GP too if you are experiencing regular headaches.

3. *Migraine aura* - These auras are relatively common and diverse in nature. Auras are visual disturbances ranging from coloured zigzag patterns, tunnel vision, moving blurred patch, to whizzing balls and so on. They last for different lengths of time depending on the individual, and

may or may not come with headaches of some description.

New migraine sufferers with auras often come in alarmed by the strangeness of the visual disturbances they have witnessed, and often this is before they are aware that they are experiencing a migraine. Auras are neurological in origin so do not result from changes to the back of the eye or any other visible sign. From listening to your symptoms and testing for sight-related causes, your optician will have a good idea of whether it is likely to be migraine auras you are experiencing.

4. *Trauma* - This is any kind of injury inflicted on the eye from blows to the eye with objects, or quite commonly with fists. Very serious cases do not tend to come to optical practices, but often people have knocks to the eye with blunt objects, causing mild red eyes or discomfort. The important thing that your optician will do is to examine your sight to make sure it is what it should be, and then to examine your eyes for scratches or damage on the outside and inside too.

    A great way of looking at the surface of the eye for scratching is with a special dye that your optician puts into the eye, and using a blue light on the microscope; any areas of damage soak up the dye and stand out to be seen with the blue light on the microscope. This dye doesn't hurt at all and doesn't affect your vision.

5. *Contact lens associated* - Modern contact lens technology and hygiene regimen mean that serious contact lens problems such as infections are now very rare, although these are still seen periodically. Most of the problems with contact lenses are due to our modern lifestyle of heavy computer use and the need to be everywhere quickly. So,

as a result, drying out of lenses resulting in dry patches on the eye is common. This is a minor issue though, usually resolved with advice or changing lenses to an alternative brand.

It is also relatively common to come across people worried about their red eyes resulting from over-wear of their contact lenses. If this is a regular problem for you then changing your lenses to more breathable lenses that will allow all-day wear is the only safe option to prevent irreversible damage to your eyes. Speak with your optician about the options.

These are just a few things that are commonplace but remember that there are many things that can affect your eyes leading to problems. They are not necessarily age-specific either; some things are just more or less common in different age groups. Your role in the eye test is to be honest and open about your sight and any concerns you may have. Your role outside of the eye test is to be aware of any problems with your sight and seek help from your optician or GP at the earliest opportunity.

20s-30s FAQs

1. *Is it possible to stop my prescription getting stronger?*

    Unfortunately there is no evidence that you can stop your prescription for glasses from changing. That is regardless of whether you are wearing them all the time or not. Some people wrongly assume that exercises are able to stop deterioration or improve your sight; that is simply not true. There is a branch of the profession which specialises in training your eyes to perform better for sports. This is very different from 'exercising your way to good sight.'

    Vision training uses scientific techniques to improve spatial awareness, hand to eye coordination and other sight-driven tasks to help improve performance. Exercises are of use if a muscle weakness exists, which is something that your optician can advise you about.

2. *I want to get my glasses and contact lenses online after my sight test, is that possible?*

    After your sight test, you are entitled to your copy of the prescription which you can use to get your glasses elsewhere if you want to. In my experience, the best opticians are geared up to give you the best experience and service – after all, it's in their interest to look after you. However, they should not make it difficult for you to make your purchase elsewhere. While not wanting to dismiss all online glasses and contact lens companies, here are some things to consider when shopping online:

Make sure the online companies can make provisions for your aftercare and can deal with any problems relating to the fit of your glasses or any other product-related issues.

Make sure the product is made to the correct standard and CE marked.

Know what country the online company is based in, and satisfy yourself that they will operate within the regulations of your home country.

If you have a moderate to high prescription, you should be extra cautious with the fitting of your glasses and lenses. In practice these often cause more complications, and usually take the expertise of a qualified dispensing optician to fit for the best results.

Because there is a cost for the service you get at your opticians, it is not possible to expect the one-to-one expert professional service, aftercare and glasses or contact lenses for next to nothing. If the professional service is less important to you, then it is totally possible to get your glasses and lenses online. I would simply advise that you make sure you are aware of what you are getting – both on and offline.

If cost is the issue, it's always worth having the discussion with your optician, and you may be surprised to find that while they may not be able to reduce their prices, they may offer you some helpful advice.

3. *Apart from my parents wearing reading glasses, neither I nor anyone in my family has eye problems, so do I need regular sight tests?*

The simple answer is yes, because you never know when problems can start. You could be the first person in your family to have a problem, you never know. For the small inconvenience of 25 minutes to get tested once every two years, you could be risking your sight.

 20s-30s Tips

If you don't have sight problems, don't get complacent about your sight, ask yourself the following questions:

1. Does anyone in my family wear glasses or have eye problems?

2. Do you drive or use computers for significant lengths of time?

3. Do you value your sight and want to keep it good?

Answering yes to any one of these questions should be a motivation to get your eyes checked every two years minimum.

2.3 THE AGE OF AWARENESS: 40s-50s

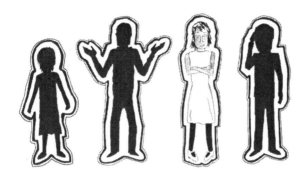

The importance of regular sight tests

The age of awareness, as I have called the 40s-50s period of life, refers to this being such a visually significant age group. Until now you may have enjoyed trouble-free sight for most of your life and never given much thought to your eyes and sight. From the age of 40 we start to notice the symptoms of failure in the normal function of our eyes that, for many, is a first reminder of how much we're all reliant on our sight.

This significant change in normal function of the eyes is due to a process called presbyopia. Presbyopia refers to the fact that the lens in the eye responsible for focusing gets less able to focus so you notice a change in your near sight for reading and other tasks. Presbyopia may well be the first awareness of significant ageing that many of us will have, because it occurs quite early in life and at a relatively young age compared with potential life expectancy.

When describing presbyopia simply, we can describe the lens in your eye as being like a disc that is fat in the middle and thin at the edges. The lens has an outer shell which is called the lens capsule. This capsule is constantly regenerating new cells all the time from birth. The old cells get pushed towards the centre of the lens and the new ones remain on the outer part of the lens.

By the time we reach about 40 the lens is getting noticeably packed full of all these old lens cells, which means it becomes harder and less flexible, so it no longer changes shape freely enough to focus things close up as well as it used to. From here on you will start to become aware of the early signs of this change as your near sight for reading starts to get worse.

"By the time we reach about 40 the lens is getting noticeably packed full..."

Age-related change

The impact of this age-related lens change can vary for different people. If you have low to moderate short-sightedness, you may find that reading books with your far sight glasses on starts to become more difficult, but reading without glasses remains perfectly fine for some time to come. If you have little or no prescription for glasses, then you are likely to find that the signs of problems with near reading start at or just over the age of 40 years.

If, on the other hand, you are someone with long-sightedness, you may be more affected than others by presbyopia and the reduced function of the lens. The reason for this is that many long-sighted individuals never need glasses before the age of 40, due to the fact that the crystalline lens in their eye still has full or good function and can work to compensate their prescription strength (see Chapter 1.4), allowing them to see well for far sight.

If their long-sightedness is not too great they may also see well for near reading without glasses below the age of 40 years. At the age of 40 or even a little earlier, your eyes start to lose this compensating ability as the lens gets harder and less flexible. You then start to find that near sight for reading becomes more blurred but, gradually, you may find that the far sight starts to become more blurred too.

So the bad news for you if you are long-sighted is that the process of presbyopia, which starts from around 40 years of age, may result in you going from never having worn glasses to needing glasses for both far and near sight by the age of 50.

This all tends to make people aware that 'your eyes are precious' as my patients often tell me at this point. I find that during the 'age of awareness', there is greater motivation to look after your eyes.

This is a good thing too, because from the age of 40 and onwards, certain eye conditions become more common, such as glaucoma. So your sight test may involve a few more tests as a matter of routine, such as measuring the pressure within your eyes and checking whether your peripheral field of vision is normal.

Mrs Spencer, a 41-year-old woman, came in for her first eye test in about four years. She has never worn glasses although records show that she has a small amount of long-sightedness and astigmatism of the following strength:

R +1.00/-0.25x15
L + 1.00/-0.25x50

Even though she is slightly long-sighted, her sight without glasses has always been better than the average good vision values of 6/6 on the sight test chart in each eye. The reason for this is simply that while the lens in her eyes had good flexibility below the age of 40, they have always been able to compensate for the effects of her long-sightedness, allowing her to still see very well.

She is now concerned about her sight, and is reporting that her eyes go a little blurred with reading after some time. It tends to be worse when tired or in low or artificial light. She finds it easier to see by holding her reading material a little further away, which is an annoyance to her. She reports that her far sight is fine on the whole, although it doesn't seem as sharp as it used to be for night driving.

Another thing that came up in the test was the fact that her father was diagnosed with glaucoma in the last year or two. With the changes to her previously reliable sight and her father having glaucoma, Mrs Spencer, a self-confessed naturally anxious woman and disliker of eye tests, was understandably quite worried. The eye test results showed that her new prescription had not changed much from four years ago:

R +1.00   Reading ADD +1.00
L + 1.25/-0.25x60   Reading ADD +1.00

Although her main prescription had not changed much, she was not seeing quite as well as she was four years ago without glasses. This time she was only able to see down to average good vision of 6/6 in each eye, just about but no better. So this explains her awareness that her sight is not as clear as it used to be for far sight, especially in night conditions because you need better sight to see optimally in low light.

The main change to be found was the reading addition of +1.00 in each eye. This is the reading strength to be added to the main prescription in each eye to make reading easier closer up. Mrs Spencer's problems were due to her having now reached the point of presbyopia. It is only at an early stage but the use of glasses for reading at this stage would mean that her eyes could stay more relaxed when reading or working up close and the glasses would do the focusing for her.

This will eliminate the symptoms of overwork such as the tired and blurred sight felt by the eyes as they try to focus the now hardening lens in the eye. This hardening lens in the eye is now also responsible for her far sight not being as sharp as it used to be, since it is now harder and doesn't flex as easily as it used to. It then struggles to compensate for Mrs Spencer's far sight and near sight.

The changes are only at the very early stages and may not need glasses just yet depending on how much a person is struggling with their sight. Things will definitely get worse for Mrs Spencer, with her far sight likely to get about two to three lines worse on the chart and her near sight likely to get about an additional 60% worse over the next 15-20 years.

Given her family history of glaucoma, Mrs Spencer would be tested for signs of it, due to the fact that glaucoma can be passed down in the family. The test results show no signs of glaucoma, which is great news for her, and she will be required to have her eyes tested yearly from now on.

Mrs Spencer's case is typical of the reluctant patient who has no problems so stays away. However, changes to her sight triggered an awareness of something being wrong and, crucially, an awareness of the importance of good sight.

Visual trends amongst the group and their possible problems

The 40s-50s age group is probably the one which places the most demand on their sight for significant lengths of time in the most diverse situations. They are unique in that if you fall within this age group, you may well be old enough to have worked through the transition from the paper-only to the digital environment. You probably spend significant time driving to and from work and you probably come home to young or teenage kids.

So your typical day involves setting off early through traffic in a 30-minute commute to work, spending several hours reading and watching things, using computers and so on. When you leave work, it's the same commute back except that it's in the opposite direction and your eyes are more tired, more sensitive and you may be driving back in lower light conditions. When you get home, it's dinner, read to the kids, watch some television, do some things on the computer and... I think you get the point.

It's a time in life when many have significant responsibilities and reliance on the vision they have been used to in their 30s. The heavy emphasis your lifestyle places on reading, watching digital displays like satellite navigation, mobile phones and computers may all highlight any flaws in your normal focusing close up, causing eye strain. If you have to do these activities then do make sure your glasses or contact lenses are up to the job and get advice from your optician about whether you are working within the range and limit of your glasses.

Many people struggle on, using glasses that are not appropriate for the task they want to use them for. Fortunately, the consequence of eye strain is nothing more than discomfort, but if left it can make viewing your task so uncomfortable that it then becomes unbearable due to the discomfort and headaches that may result. Due to the widely varying nature of the task that you may find yourself doing throughout the day, a multifocal pair of glasses may prove to be the most convenient solution to your problems.

"Many people struggle on, using glasses that are not appropriate for the task they want to use them for."

Varifocal lenses may prove to be the most versatile option as far as glasses go, offering the benefit of far, medium and near range sight all combined into one pair of glasses. There is a misconception that having varifocal, or bifocal glasses for that matter, means you have to wear them all the time. That is not true, because the benefit of them is that you will have all the clarity you need in one pair of glasses for convenience instead of two or three pairs of glasses.

When you have finished the task that you need them for, you can take them off if you wish, you can use them as and when you need, based on your optician's advice. The best method of correcting your sight for best convenience will be different from individual to individual and will depend on the exact nature of what you will be using them for and in what kind of environment.

Five common conditions affecting this age group

1. *Glaucoma* - This can be thought of in simple terms as the situation when the pressure inside the eyeball becomes too high, damaging the back of the eye – a bit like blowing up a balloon so much that it starts to damage the wall of the balloon. It usually affects one eye first and is most common from the age of 40 onwards. The result of glaucoma is that the cells of the retina start to die off gradually from the edges of your vision inwards to the centre.

The most common form of glaucoma is very slow to develop, over some years usually, and has no signs to look out for, so you can't expect to feel high pressure or anything like that. The only effective way of catching glaucoma early is through regular eye tests. Your optician has several ways of determining whether you may have the signs of glaucoma.

The three common tests at their disposal are looking through to the back of your eye, checking your field of vision for damage and measuring the pressure inside your eye. If there is any chance that you may have glaucoma, you will be referred for confirmation by the hospital eye department.

The bad news is that glaucoma is one of the leading causes of preventable blindness because people fail to get their eyes tested regularly. The good news, however, is that it never has to cause you a problem if it is detected early and treated. Treatment is simply, in most cases, regular drops in the eye to bring the pressure down to a healthy level.

2. *Floaters* - Describes the presence of particles in the vitreous gel floating about in your sight. They are most noticeable against a bright white background, such as when you are looking up at the sky. They are due to the normally solid vitreous gel in the eye degenerating and contracting, which then results in it becoming more of a mobile gel. Dark fibres may then collect in the gel forming 'floaters' of different sizes.

Floaters do not go away, but if they're quite large, they may get broken up with time, making them less noticeable. Floaters on their own do not require treatment, but they do need investigation by your optician as soon as possible when you first get them, and this is especially true if you are experiencing flashes of light too. Your optician will want to check to make sure there is no sign of retinal tears or detachments of any type at the back of your eyes and may well refer you to the local hospital eye department for further investigation.

Floaters are very common and while more commonly associated with age, younger people can get them too, particularly if they get regular blows to the head playing sports like boxing or football. They are usually present as just a few floaters, so if you experience a sudden shower of them, this may point to a retinal detachment. Retinal detachments need urgent attention, so either call your optician for advice first or go straight to a local hospital eye department for investigation.

3. *PVD* - Stands for posterior vitreous detachment. The vitreous gel in the eye is contained in a transparent sack, a bit like cling film, known as the posterior vitreous. This sack is held in two places, the circle ring to the front entrance of the eye and a smaller ring out to the back exit of the eye. It is part of this posterior ring that can become detached from the back resulting in a ring-like floater or cobweb-like floater reported by many.

It is not unusual for people to report flashes of light before noticing this sudden large floater. The flashing occurs when the transparent sack rattles; you may then experience the flash in the outer corner of your sight. The causes include age, blows to the head and high short-sightedness. Treatment is only needed if tears in the 'cling film' sack or the retina are detected, to prevent sight damage through retinal detachment. Otherwise it does not cause a problem and just needs monitoring at your normal eye tests.

4. *Retinal detachments* - As the name suggests, this is the situation where the retina, the eye's light-sensitive layer, comes off. This then needs urgent surgery to attempt to put it back in place, and hopefully save as much of the sight as possible. Although it can happen to anyone regardless of age, retinal detachments are most common in people with high short-sightedness or those who regularly get blows to the head, such as boxers.

Symptoms include a sudden presence of lots of floating dust like particles in your sight, flashing lights and loss of sight appearing as a curtain over the affected eye. Your optician will check your sight for comparison with your previous visits or comparison with your other eye. The examination of the back of your eye will show exactly what's going on. You will then be sent directly down to the local hospital eye casualty department.

If you suspect you have retinal detachment, you would be best heading directly down to a hospital eye casualty department, because early treatment right away could save your sight. More often than not, a suspected retinal detachment may just turn out to be normal floaters or PVD, which require investigation but no treatment.

5. *Blepharitis* - This is the inflammation of the eyelid margins, leaving them looking red with flaking skin along their margins. There may also be some redness of the white of the eye along with itching or aching. The cause is often bacterial infection at the root of the eyelashes, sometimes resulting in repeated conjunctivitis. It is often found later in life, but can also be more common in those with allergy or sensitive skin conditions such as eczema.

Treatment in most cases is managing the condition with good eyelid hygiene. The usual advice is to keep the eyelid margins clean using diluted baby shampoo, because it is non-irritant, on a cotton bud and use it to clean the eyelid and eyelash region gently but thoroughly. You can also buy specially formulated eyelid scrub products available on the market. Keeping the eyelid margins clean and clear of flakes is the key to managing the condition and stopping recurrent bacterial infections. As long as you are doing this, your eyes should remain relatively comfortable.

40s-50s FAQs

1. *What are the early signs of near sight reading problems?*

    You may notice one or all of the following signs or symptoms at or near the age of 40 years:

    - Having to hold reading material further away for better clarity.

    - Sight is more blurred when tired.

    - Near sight for reading is harder in low or artificial light.

    - Focusing takes more time, especially after reading for some time or when tired.

2. *Will my near sight reading problems get worse?*

    Unfortunately yes, reading will become more difficult. Once the process starts, it deteriorates quite quickly at the beginning, slows down, then comes to a point where it stays stable and eventually stops. At this point you will find that reading anything at near sight is almost impossible without your glasses.

3. *What is the solution to near sight reading problems?*

    When the symptoms start affecting your ability to read or work in comfort, glasses are advisable. No amount of exercising the eye or struggling on without glasses is going to help reverse the situation. The use of glasses will put your eyes at ease by letting the glasses do much of the focusing so that your eyes can be more relaxed.

 40s-50s Tips

Have you considered contact lenses as a solution to your reading problem? You may be suitable for multifocal contact lenses that correct both far and near sight in one. While not everyone is suited to these, those who are often experience an amazing sense of freedom.

It's not too late to start wearing contact lenses.

2.4 THE AGE OF DEGENERATION: 60s+

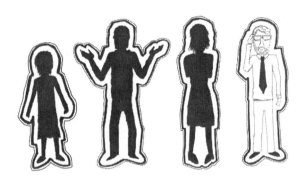

The importance of regular sight tests

I come across many over-60s who have good vision and are far from the shy, retiring people we sometimes stereotype them to be. However, as much as we hope that our eyes go on looking and seeing well in the same way that they may have done for years, the reality is that the ageing process really starts to set in from 60 years and onwards. The hallmark of this is the increased occurrence of eye disease and age-related eye conditions in the over-60 years category.

It really isn't as gloomy as it sounds though; the eye has an amazing propensity to look after itself, but at this stage in life it requires a little more attention and monitoring to maintain the optimum sight and performance your eye is capable of.

Age-related change

Many things about our eyes change with age, and many of my patients often come to see me with concerns over changes in their eyes, which are often down to the ageing process. These changes rarely require any treatment at all but my observation is that, out of fear, many over 60-year-olds avoid coming in to be tested for fear of getting bad news.

Here I will highlight some of the most common age-related changes with the eye that you should be aware of. Many people find it reassuring to know that some things can be put down to age rather than disease. The diagram in the 'Know your way around the eye' chapter may be a helpful reference for you here.

Eyelids - With age, the skin of the eyelids will become loose to varying degrees between individuals. For some it may be minimal, while for others it may sag in a cosmetically noticeable way. The muscles within the lids that control blinking may also be affected, causing a loss of strength. The result may be drooping top eyelids or rolling in or out of the lower eyelid. In some cases these eyelid muscle degenerations may require surgical treatment. This is a decision you will have to discuss with your optician or eye surgeon.

Eyelashes - You can expect fewer lashes with age due to degeneration of the lash follicles.

Tears - Dry eye tends to be more common with age for several reasons. The older you are, the more likely you are to be on medications, and some of these may contribute to dryness of the eyes. Another reason for dry eyes, however, could be that with age your tears may reduce in quality. This reduction can be due to the degeneration in function of the pores and glands that release the different parts of your tears, making them less efficient.

Conjunctiva - With age and exposure to UV light over the years, this normally transparent layer over the white of the eye tends to become thicker and less transparent. As a result you may find yellowing raised areas called pinguecula, usually on the part of the white of the eye nearest to the nose on both eyes. These raised, slightly yellow or white areas vary in appearance but do not usually need any treatment, and may change very slowly over time. Mention it to your optician at your next appointment to confirm that it is normal.

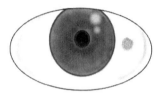

Pinguecula (Right Eye)

Sclera - The white of the eye may start to lose some of its whiteness with age and may even become thin in places. Thinning of the white reveals a darker patch of blue-black coloured layer underneath. This causes no problem and does not need treatment.

Cornea - Often develops a white ring or partial ring called arcus senilis out towards its edge. These rings are not unusual with age and can sometimes be linked with having a high fat content diet at some period of life.

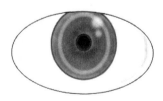

Arcus Senilis

Iris - One of the obvious changes to the iris relates to the muscles within it that control your pupil size by contracting or relaxing. Degeneration of these muscles with age may result in smaller and less responsive pupils. This isn't much of a problem and in fact smaller pupils can make seeing easier in some situations, such as when you are out in the sunshine.

The Lens - As described earlier, the crystalline lens is constantly regenerating its outer layer of cells, and pushing the old layers to the centre. This means that the lens will eventually become so packed full that it can't flex at all to focus for near sight reading. This packing full of the lens also has the effect of making the lens less transparent, contributing to cataract development. Cataract has many causes, but the most common cause is normal ageing. This will result in glare problems, difficulty reading in low light and so on.

Vitreous gel - With age the vitreous gel degenerates and contracts, becoming more liquid, making things like floating particles in the gel more common with age.

Retina - Many of the age-related changes in the retina affect its function. So you may find things like your eyes taking longer to recover from bright lights or longer to adapt to dark light conditions. The cause of these types of problems may be due to the reduction in efficiency of the chemical reaction in the cells of the retina, making them slower to respond to the light.

Macula - This is the central part of the retina responsible for the sharp detail we all rely on for recognising faces, seeing text on television and reading. General changes at the macula will be the same as that of the rest of the retina, but one of the most common changes that can develop here is age-related macular degeneration, affecting the quality of your central vision.

Vessels - The effect of ageing on the vessels of the eye is the same for that throughout the whole body. The vessels tend to lose their elasticity and may even become narrower in conditions such as arteriosclerosis (hardening of the arteries).

Muscles - With age there may be a general loss of muscle tone in all the muscles of the eye and lids, due to normal age-related degeneration. The eyes continue to stay mobile and blinking remains, although there will be an inevitable loss of responsiveness compared to the young eye.

If you are concerned about any changes of the eye, always seek medical advice.

Some of the practical ways in which age can affect you from 60 years and beyond can be highlighted as we examine the following case of a gentleman that I had dealt with in practice.

Mr Graham, a 69-year-old gentleman with a great passion for reading, came for his regular eye test, reporting increased frustration at not being able to read as well as he'd like. Over the years, he has accumulated a collection of over 2,500 books on local history and other diverse interests. He now finds himself in the situation of not being able to read many of his books comfortably.

Other problems reported include a gritty, aching feeling in the eyes that is worse with reading despite using artificial tear drops and, his wife reports, a white ring round the edge of the coloured part of the eye. From a medical point of view Mr Graham has been treated for arthritis, high blood pressure and cholesterol by his GP for the last 15 years or so.

On examination, Mr Graham was found to have reduced sight even through the best glasses possible for his eyes. His sight on the test chart was found to be 6/18 in the right eye and 6/24 in the left eye, which represents five lines worse in the right eye than average good sight and about six lines worse in the left eye. The cause of this reduction in sight was down to two issues in the eye.

Firstly Mr Graham was found to have significant cataract in both eyes making it difficult to look through to the back of his eyes. Drops to make his pupils bigger in order to look through the cataract better were put into his eyes and a more detailed examination of the front and back of his eyes was carried out with the microscope.

The surface of the eye shows age-related changes and the signs of dry eye, evident by assessing his tear quality with the dye test. Internally, behind the cataract there is evidence of early dry macular degeneration in the left eye but no evidence of any in the right eye.

Given the extent of cataract and the presence of early dry macular degeneration, Mr Graham is advised that referral for cataract removal is the best course of action before glasses would be of any benefit. He is advised that the white ring on the coloured part of his eye is age-related and may be linked to his previous cholesterol problems. The gritty eyes are due to dry eyes which is more common in people with arthritic conditions, and some of the medications that he is being treated with may contribute to dry eyes too.

This is nothing to worry about and the medications he is on are doing him good. I recommend lubricating eye drops for him to use to remedy the grittiness and aching. About three months later, following surgical treatment, I see Mr Graham again to find that he has now had the cataract removed from both eyes, although I had warned him that the surgeons may advise against surgery in the left eye if they felt that the vision would not be any better due to the macular degeneration, or if they were worried about the risk of disturbing it, making things worse quicker.

Having retested his sight, the results were significantly improved, with his right eye now able to see to the average good sight line of 6/6 while the left eye was improved down to 6/9. He was delighted with the result, and new glasses ensured that he was back to reading significantly better.

We discussed the future prospects for his sight, in particular the likely deterioration of his macular degeneration and the benefits of the eye supplement tablets that he was prescribed by the surgeon. He also informs me that his eyes now have longer-lasting comfort with the lubricant drops compared to the artificial tears that he used to use.

Visual trends amongst this group

In the over-60 age category the prevailing trend is the continued desire to read printed books as well as the other near sight reliant activities such as knitting and puzzles. The reading of books is by no means a phenomenon that is on the way out in the younger generation, but with the luxury of more free time in retirement, reading is understandably a favourite pastime of the over-60s.

For many in or approaching retirement, they have grown up without all the technological distractions to reading faced by this generation, so the idea of retirement still conjures up the image of relaxing with a book. The interesting thing is that, once in retirement, some people find that their near sight for reading is compromised by age, disease or health-related factors.

" ...I have noticed a growing trend in the over-60s using devices such as handheld game devices and tablet computers... "

Contrary to the idea that all over-60s are technology shy, I have noticed a growing trend in the over-60s using devices such as handheld game devices and tablet computers to play games, solve puzzles and, increasingly, to read. These and other such devices have the advantage of being versatile and adaptable to your level of sight. They are also very instinctive and simple enough to use that it opens up the huge possibilities and advantages for dealing better with some of the problems faced by the ageing eye.

These problems include contrast, brightness, font style and size issues, which can now be adjusted to suit the individual. As electronic reading resources become more accessible to every budget, the benefit to more mature eyes will increase as the technologies are optimised for the retired consumer.

Five common conditions affecting the 60+ age group

1 *Cataract* - This is the situation where the crystalline lens in the eye develops thick patches blocking or disrupting the passage of light through to the back of the eye. There can be several causes of cataract such as diabetes, long-term use of high-dose steroids, trauma and so on. These tend to bring on cataract earlier in life whereas ageing causes cataract later in life.

There is a normal loss of clarity of this lens with age, causing it to appear more brown in colour as it absorbs some of the light that it used to let through, but it may never develop into a full cataract. The point where the normal loss of clarity of the lens is described as a cataract is not always obvious. As a guide, when it affects your vision in any way then we can be certain in calling it a cataract.

The problems caused by cataracts are obvious in that they simply make it more difficult to see because it becomes more like looking through a frosted bathroom window. They do not need treatment until they make a noticeable impact on your sight or lifestyle and you want them treated. Until this point, many surgeons may not advise treatment.

For this reason some opticians choose not to alarm their patients in the early stages of the lens going cloudy due to normal ageing by announcing that a 'cataract is forming' prematurely. When the time is right, it will usually require a referral from your optician for assessment by a surgeon, who can then treat the cataract by removing it surgically. Cataract extraction operations are one of the most successful yet dramatically life-enhancing operations that you can have done.

2 *AMD* - Age-related macular degeneration, also sometimes abbreviated to ARMD. It is the result of age-related disruption of deep vessels below the macula, which causes them to leak some of their content. This then results in yellow deposits (Dry AMD) in the macula causing gradual reduction of central sight. Worse cases result in bleeding (Wet AMD) into the macula causing sudden damage to the central sight.

The dry type of AMD is far more common and although both types can eventually lead to central sight loss, the dry AMD progresses over years rather than hours and days, as may be the case with the wet type. Peripheral sight will not be affected so total sight loss will not take place.

At the moment there is no treatment for dry AMD and no permanent treatment for wet AMD. The current best treatment for wet AMD is a drug called Lucentis (Ranibizumab), which has been shown to stop wet AMD getting worse or significantly slow down the rate and impact of deterioration. The title 'age-related' makes AMD sound like something that we are all destined to get because of age, but the good news is that it will not affect the vast majority of people.

3 *Hypertensive (high blood pressure) eye disease* - Long-term uncontrolled hypertension, or high blood pressure as it is commonly known, can cause damage to the blood vessels gradually over time. This results in increased risk of strokes and burst blood vessels in the eye due to blockages of the vessels where they narrow.

When your optician examines the back of your eye we can often see the result of long-term uncontrolled high blood pressure on the blood vessels of the eye. The affected vessels tend to look more bent and distorted in size. In extreme cases of uncontrolled blood pressure, damage may progress to cause leaking or burst blood vessels. This then poses the risk of significant loss of sight.

Your optician will examine your eyes for any signs needing medical or surgical intervention. Regaining control of your blood pressure through an improved diet, lifestyle and medication, according to the advice of your doctor, can reverse some of the signs of blood vessel damage mentioned.

4 *Diabetic eye disease* - Diabetes is a common condition causing blood sugar levels to become too high. It can be

managed well with medication and diet, but long term it has the problem of damaging the small blood vessels throughout the body, including the eye.

With time or bad control of your blood sugar, the small vessels in the eye become damaged by the high sugar levels, causing them to leak. This happens throughout the body, but in the eye the effects of this can be observed, giving your optician or doctor an indication of how the body is being affected. We grade the stage of diabetic eye disease based on how much blood is leaking, what other materials are leaking and the location of the leak.

The most urgent threat is if the centre of the sight is at risk through bleeding at the part of the retina called the macula. Apart from that, other areas of bleeding may be present as little bleed spots that won't affect the sight in any significant way, so do not need treatment. Treatment for bleeds is usually with laser to seal them and then good control of the blood sugar is essential through advice from your doctor.

Diabetes does make you more at risk of fluctuating sight and other eye conditions, so more frequent eye tests than average are required to prevent other problems sneaking up on you unknowingly, such as glaucoma. Good blood sugar control is key to prevention of diabetic eye disease.

5 *Watery eyes* - This is a huge cause of annoyance to many sufferers. It can result in dry eye, strangely enough, due to the fact that because the tears are streaming down the face instead of covering and lubricating the eye, the surface may start to experience drying out. The reasons for watery eyes can be one or a combination of several things. Your tears have three layers: oil on the outside, water in the middle and mucus on the innermost layer touching the eye.

The function of the mucus is to hold the water and oil on the eye, so if production or release of the mucus layer is low, it can lead to the tears not staying on the eye as they should. However, this may not account for a lot of the tears running off the eye. Other reasons that could explain this would be either overactive water glands, full or partial blockage of the passage that the tears drain through or the lower eyelid rolling either inwards or outwards, causing tears to run off the eyelid. Any one of these conditions could result in tears streaming down the face regularly.

Your optician will be able to tell you what the likely cause may be in your case and advise you of what can be done. Treatment will depend on which condition is causing your watery eye. Drainage blockage may require a simple procedure to open up the drainage passage which can narrow or block with age. Eyelids that roll in or out will require surgery to fix and any indication of overactive tear production would need further investigation at a hospital eye department. Fortunately most cases of watery eyes are not serious and will not damage your sight.

60s+ FAQs

1. *My eyes keep watering but my optician says I have dry eyes?*

   Simply put, any situation that results in tears running off the eye instead of staying on to keep it moist may result in dryness of the eye. It may seem illogical, but you need the tears to stay on the eye long enough to protect them, particularly in situations where you are concentrating and staring a lot because the eyes become more exposed to the air making it more likely that your eyes dry out as the exposed tears evaporate quicker.

2. *Is it true that arthritis can affect my eyes?*

   Arthritis is a very common condition in the elderly population. It can be caused when immune system cells which normally protect you start to attack your joints and body. Arthritis can be linked to dry eye and inflammatory conditions of the eye such as iritis. Consult your optician or doctor about any specific problems you are having

3. *Why do you need to know about all the medications I am taking?*

   Sometimes people withhold medical information because they do not feel it is relevant to their eyes. It may or may not be relevant but bear in mind that it can be linked to some eye problems you may be having or can explain some signs that your optician is seeing.

Some drugs cause signs of toxicity in the eye, early cataracts, or make you more prone to rarer infections if they reduce the activity of your immune system, and so on. These are all things your optician will have to look out for.

 60s+ Tips

Reading for significant lengths of time should be done using good, even lighting without shadows being cast on the book you are reading, for the best visual comfort. The light should be as near to average daylight as possible, which means using a whiter light rather than the yellow light produced by standard or fluorescent bulbs.

This poorer quality yellow light doesn't make it to the back of the eye so easily if you have an early cataract or normal hazing of the lens in your eye, which is very common from the age of 60 years onwards. This then makes it harder to read and see lower contrast objects. Bright and whiter light gets to the back of the eye better, resulting in better clarity all round.

If you have relatively low vision, enjoy reading but have been struggling with paper-based reading material, consider trying an electronic device. With many of these devices you may find reading much easier, with better contrast and the ability to make the text bigger and brighter. Make sure you get a demonstration first before you buy any such device.

3. MAKE IT MAXIMUM

Maximum sight is the best sight that your eyes are capable of if perfect optical conditions exist, allowing light to focus cleanly on the light-sensitive cells of the retina at the back of the eye. Your maximum may be different from someone else's depending on whether the resolution of your retina cells has developed normally from childhood. Whatever maximum you have, it is important to benefit from it and look after it.

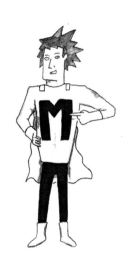

I'm always amazed when people knowingly choose to continue without any sight correction for driving or other tasks after they are shown how poor their sight is without glasses compared to how great it could be with glasses. This is often out of a misguided belief that they are 'seeing well enough' or they are 'strengthening their eyes' and occasionally it is just for cosmetic reasons.

On the other hand there are those with poor sight that can't be helped at all by glasses or any other corrective measure. These individuals would do practically anything to have a little bit of extra sight if it was available to them. It appears so often to be true that good sight is something only fully appreciated by those who don't have access to it.

The challenge to the eye care profession is to better educate the nation about how best to look after your sight in the good times, when everything may be going well, so that you stand a better chance of good sight in retirement and beyond. With more of us living longer and longer, the question of whether your sight will 'see you through' is more important now than ever.

The process of looking after your sight involves maintaining and making the most of the sight that you have. It's my observation that always making sure you have as good a vision as possible with glasses or contact lenses helps you to be more sensitive and aware of subtle deterioration to your sight, which may then ring alarm bells that prompt you to get your eyes checked earlier.

This can potentially save your sight if acting fast and seeking attention early means that a sight-threatening condition is treated before it causes a problem. If you are someone avoiding wearing glasses and putting up with less clarity than your eye is capable of, then you may find that you won't notice further blurring of your sight quite as easily as you would if your vision was as sharp as possible.

"It appears so often to be true that good sight is something only fully appreciated by those who don't have access to it."

Your sight in the future can be affected by the things you do now, when things may be much clearer. Here I highlight five key factors affecting maximum sight, and how to ensure it remains maximum for as long as possible.

#1 CHOOSE YOUR LENSES CAREFULLY

In the first chapter I said that if the eyes were the window to the soul, then your optician can be thought of as the window cleaner. I also mentioned that there are two types of optician that have to be qualified and registered to provide professional services to you. I have talked primarily from the viewpoint of the optician that does the eye test.

The other optician that is often overlooked is the dispensing optician. Their training is in giving you optimum sight out of your glasses, through expert optical knowledge and up-to-date product knowledge. Optical assistants can be trained in-house to do some of the basics, but fundamentally, without at least one dispensing optician supervising their work, you could have the best eye test in the world only to have some of that ruined by poor advice outside the test room.

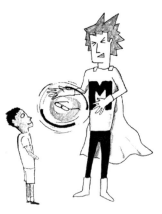

Eyewear is a significant investment to your sight. The quality of the advice you get regarding the best products for your eyes is critical. Although optical assistants may be adequately trained to deal with the average case, they are not experts so should really be supervised by a dispensing optician. Here are some of the ways of achieving optimum clarity that your dispensing optician may talk to you about.

Get thinner lenses

If you have a high prescription of -6.00 for example, you will be aware that your glasses are likely to have thick edges. This motivates you to have a high index thin lens, but instead of going for the thinnest lens you can afford, you opt for a little bit less because you don't think it will make any significant difference to the thickness of the lenses. That is a fair point, but the benefits of thinner lenses go beyond the cosmetic look of your glasses.

Thinner lenses offer several optical advantages over the thicker alternatives. A thick lens edge allows more light to bounce within the lens, causing more glare to obstruct your view, making it more difficult to see in certain conditions. The other issue caused by internal reflections within a thicker lens is the phenomenon known as power rings. Power rings are multiple ring images of your eye seen by others looking at you while you're wearing your glasses.

Thick lenses can also make your eye appear bigger if you are long-sighted or smaller if you are short-sighted. All these optical features of the thicker lens can be reduced significantly or eliminated by the use of high index lenses to make the lenses appear thinner. Long-sighted lenses have a thicker centre, so to make them thinner it is best achieved by also making them flatter at the front with aspheric lenses. Aspheric lenses are ones that have a flatter curvature towards the edge.

With the thinnest and flattest lenses available, light has less room to bounce about inside the lens, improving the clarity of view through the lenses in high or low light levels. The problem of power rings can also be resolved by thinning the lenses. This makes the size of your eye when others look at you appear more normal through the lens too. So thinner and flatter lenses make optical improvements to the vision through your glasses, while making them lighter and cosmetically improved.

Optimum lens recommendations:

-   Short-sighted individuals: go for the thinnest lenses you can afford.

-   Long-sighted individuals: go for the thinnest and flattest (aspheric lens) lenses you can afford.

Cut out reflections

Optimum clarity requires as much light getting through to your eye as possible. When you look into a mirror, you do not see through to the other side of the glass, but rather you see everything that is in front of the mirror including yourself. This is because mirrors generally reflect 100% of the light hitting its surface back to our eyes through the process of reflection.

In the same respect, if your glasses lens was reflecting 100% of the light hitting it, it would become a mirror and no one looking at you would be able to see your eyes and you would not be able to see through the lenses because 0% of the light is passing through the lens to your eye. While that sounds extreme, the reality is that an element of this will be going on with standard lenses on your glasses.

Each surface of a plastic lens reflects 8% of the light hitting its surface, and since the lens has a front and back surface, that means up to 16% of light will be reflected off the surface of each lens in each eye. That means that 16% of the light may not get to your eye, reducing the visibility of your eye to onlookers, and reducing the quality of what you can see through your lenses.

The other issue arising from all this reflected light coming off the surfaces of your lens is that it creates a constant mist of all this reflected light in front of you which then adds to creating ghosting or halos around the image you are looking at. This is the problem that anti-reflection coatings aim to solve.

Anti-reflection or MAR (multiple anti-reflection) coating works by cutting the 8% reflection to just 1% off each surface, resulting in up to 2% loss due to reflection from your glasses' lenses instead of 16%. That is a significant improvement, which then means that when there is not much light about, the glasses are not wasting light due to reflection so clarity is improved over lenses without an anti-reflection coating.

One of the downsides of having all the reflections on the surface of the lens cut to just 1% is that fingerprints and grime on the lens surface are no longer hidden by the reflections. Many quality anti-reflection coated lenses now come with a hydrophobic coating that also makes cleaning easier.

Optimum anti-reflection lens recommendation:

- Remember anti-reflection coated lenses need more regular cleaning.

- Anti-reflection coating is great in your near sight glasses too, helping you read with less glare in low light.

Reduce steamed-up lenses

Anyone who is a wearer of glasses will be familiar with the problem of lenses steaming up – to your embarrassment or, worse still, in dangerous situations. The problem is most common when the body is giving off a lot of heat and the lens surface is relatively cool, such as during exercise. It can also be a problem in rainy, wet or foggy conditions. When moisture gets on to the lens it starts to collect and fogs the lens.

The only solution to this problem is to treat the lens with a hydrophobic coating. This coating simply makes the surface of the lens repellent to moisture so it doesn't collect on the lens but runs off the lens instead. The way hydrophobic lens coatings are often sold in optical practices may make them appear to be a luxury, but in some situations, particularly sports and driving, they may prove to be essential in maintaining clarity and safety.

Reduce glare through polarising lenses

Polarising lenses have a particular benefit in environments where there is a lot of light scattered causing glare, preventing you from seeing what you are doing. Fishing is a classic example of an environment when your optimum sight can be greatly reduced by the reflections off the surface of the water. Light hits the water and reflects off in many different directions, resulting in a dazzling effect that we call glare. Polarised lenses work by filtering out much of the multi-directional scattered light that causes dazzle.

The result is that you have one directional light getting to your eye, making it less dazzling and clearer for your eyes to see detail in objects. There are many other conditions in which polarised lenses can be used. They do have a natural light tint on them so for safety reasons they are not advisable for night driving

Tips

Many of the medium to premium lenses will come with multiple anti-reflection and hydrophobic coatings as standard. So when comparing the value of lenses in your glasses check whether these clarity options come included in the price. The benefit to sight and clarity with some of these lens add-ons can be significant, so make sure you are aware of the benefits before turning them down or opting not to have them on your new glasses when you have had them on your current pair.

#2 TWO KEY ENEMIES THAT MUST BE FOUGHT

The ageing process will inevitably bring a natural reduction in sight due to reducing performance of the cells of the whole body. The processes in the eye that keep the eye clear may no longer perform as efficiently as they used to, so it is normal to find that for these and other age-related reasons there may be some decline in sight with age.

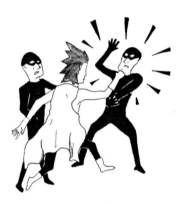

However, there are two 'enemies' which must be fought if long-term optimum sight is to be maintained. UV light exposure and smoking are two key factors that can accelerate the problems associated with ageing, contributing to potentially sight-threatening conditions. Crucially though, these two enemies can be fought.

UV light

Ultraviolet (UV) light is the invisible light radiation all around us that in high levels causes sunburn on the skin. UV from the sun is categorised into three different levels: UVA, UVB and UVC, with UVC being the most powerful and potentially harmful. Only UVA and UVB make it into our atmosphere because the ozone layer absorbs the UVC radiation. The main difference between the three types of UV can be thought of as how far it can penetrate into the cells and layers of the body, causing damage.

It is thought that UVB is the most harmful because it is capable of causing sunburn and damage to the DNA of skin cells which may lead to the development of skin cancer. UVA is thought by some to be relatively harmless because it doesn't affect the tissues of the body in a way that causes burns or direct damage to DNA in cells. However, other schools of thought suggest that UVA may be just as harmful because it is believed to cause damage to vitamins in body tissue, causing the creation and build-up of highly unstable particles called free radicals.

The damage of these vitamins means that their health benefits are lost, and the increase of free radicals can cause damage to other tissues including DNA, leading to cancers and so on. This potential risk of UVA is not one that should be overlooked, because the damage is potentially significant. So through what is a complex and scientific process to explain, there is the potential for UVA and UVB to cause problems in the external and internal eye.

The eye is designed with protective layers that are capable of absorbing low levels of these harmful UV rays, but the more intense the UV, the more problematic it can become. The damage that can be caused by UV on the outer eye ranges from arc eye (photokeratitis or welder's flash) to drying and thickening of the surface. The crystalline lens in the eye can absorb UV, but too much over a long time can cause damage to the content of the lens, resulting in early cataract. Further back into the eye, the retina can be harmed too by UV exposure.

A major condition that may arise from UV damage is age-related macular degeneration (AMD). In very simple terms,

AMD is due to age-related thickening of a deep membrane (or layer) beneath the retina, which then disrupts deep lying vessels. When this happens within the macula region of the retina, it may cause some content of the vessels to leak, damaging the macula region of the retina. UV exposure over time is also thought to contribute to this process happening early.

The benefits of protecting your eyes from harmful UV cannot be overstated, and while the eyes do a great job all on their own, the effect of UV exposure over the years can be significant, and possibly worse as the eye gets less efficient generally as a result of natural ageing.

So what can we do about this UV problem? Well, if you are a glasses wearer then the good news is that standard plastic lenses do a very good job of blocking out harmful UV light. However, they do not give full protection, leaving you still exposed to some risk. Polycarbonate plastic lenses are naturally 100% UV blocking, but apart from that the other option open to you is the use of a UV-coated lens treatment. This lens coating blocks 100% of the UV in standard glasses and sunglasses lenses.

No matter how good your lenses are at blocking the UV radiation, you will still find that you are exposed at the edges and sides of your glasses if they are a particularly narrow design or fitted too far from your face. So make sure they are well fitted and give you good coverage, looking all around out of the corner of your eyes.

Sunglasses, as I mentioned, can be a common cause of people getting arc eye or other UV exposure-related issues. There is the perception that looking through very tinted sunglasses protects you from harm, when the reality is that you may be exposing yourself to more harm if the sunglasses are not 100%

UV blocking or wrapped to fit your face closely. The reason is that behind dark tints your pupils dilate, making your eyes more vulnerable to stray UV radiation than they would be if the pupils were smaller.

Another UV blocking option is the use of photochromic lenses which are the lenses that become tinted outdoors and clear indoors. They are 100% UV blocking because the chemical reaction that causes them to change colour absorbs and reacts with UV light. However, as photochromic lenses age, the chemical reaction fades and the UV protection may become compromised.

UV levels are at their most dangerous at high altitudes, in snowy conditions and reflecting off water. Full UV protection is essential at these times especially and a constant and dark tint is advisable for dealing with the light intensity.

"There is the perception that looking through very tinted sunglasses protects you from harm, when the reality is that you may be exposing yourself to more harm if the sunglasses are not 100% UV blocking..."

Smoking

Smoking is an example of a lifestyle choice that affects the whole body, including the eye, in a destructive way. Cigarettes contain a whole host of toxic substances that have the potential to do serious harm if you are a smoker. Many of these substances, once in your system, can cause gradual damage of internal organs and tissue by a range of mechanisms, many not fully understood.

The main way for many of these toxins to travel throughout the body is in the bloodstream from the lungs. Over the years, these toxic materials start to damage the blood vessels, increasing the risk of high blood pressure, hardening of the arteries, heart attacks, strokes and so on. Within the eye, smoking can increase the risk of macular degeneration as it damages the vessels underneath the macula, causing them to leak.

Other effects on vision include the development of earlier cataracts and optic nerve problems. Because smoking is linked to other conditions such as high blood pressure, you then have to contend with the eye problems that these secondary conditions may cause in the eye. Smokers may experience external redness of the eye due to irritation of the eyes as they are irritated by some of the toxic substances in the cigarettes.

Passive smoking will also result in the same problems, so children or anyone in a shared house should be protected from inhaling cigarette smoke.

Tips

- Wear 100% UV blocking lenses such as polycarbonate, photochromic or get a UV coating added to the lens in your everyday glasses.

- Sunglasses must be 100% UV blocking or 'UV 400' marked.

- Slightly yellow-tinted driving lenses can block harmful UV radiation.

- Children wearing toy sunglasses out in the sun can be at risk. Use only full UV blocking sunglasses.

- Wearing hats and visors to shield yourself from UV is thought to reduce the likelihood of UV-related eye conditions such as AMD and cataract.

- Quit smoking to help reduce some of the effects and damage it causes to the retina. Smoking contributes to damage of the pigmented layer of the retina which leads to degeneration of the retinal cells.

#3 EATING FOR YOUR SIGHT

The popular saying 'you are what you eat' hints to the fact that what we eat affects our whole body, but it also carries many truths about the eye in as far as healthy eating can help combat health-related sight problems. Health problems can result when cells lack the nutrients they need to maintain their normal processes and functions. Other nutrients can have protective effects, keeping harmful processes at bay.

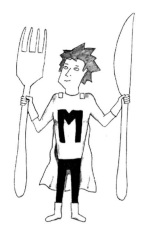

The biggest problem faced by today's 'high speed everything' society is that our diets may be limited by what we can get on the go or prepare conveniently. Cost is also another factor which determines what we eat in times of rising costs and squeezed budgets. However, a diet that is balanced is key to long-term healthy sight. Here we will now look at some of the main nutrients that are essential for optimum sight, where they are found and how they help the sight.

Antioxidants

Antioxidants are very important substances for the health and well-being of the whole body, primarily because of their ability to deal with and 'mop up' harmful free radicals. Free radicals are highly charged and unstable particles created by the process of oxidation in cells, which happens normally in the body. Free radicals go whizzing about causing damage to other particles in cells, making them unstable too, or damaging their DNA, which can lead to mutations resulting in cancers or abnormalities.

Antioxidants are able to make free radicals stable by undoing the oxidation process that caused them, making free radicals harmless. The three Vitamins A, C and E are all antioxidants; here are the foods that you can find them present in.

Vitamin A: Is important for night vision. It is needed by the cells of the retina to make the chemical needed to react with light and create the visual signal for sight. Without enough of it, your sight would take longer to clear coming from bright light into dark conditions, and overall you would experience poorer sight in low light levels. It may also be helpful with some dry eye conditions.

Foods containing Vitamin A: Cod liver oil, butter, eggs, milk, beef or chicken livers.

Vitamin C: Is thought to have benefits in reducing the impact of macular degeneration and the formation of cataract. Like other antioxidants, Vitamin C can mop up free radical particles that may play a part in damaging deep vessels in the macula, responsible for macular degeneration formation.

Foods containing Vitamin C: Strawberries, red or green sweet peppers, oranges, broccoli.

Vitamin E: In combination with antioxidants, Vitamin C and a type of Vitamin A may reduce the progression to advanced macular degeneration.

Foods containing Vitamin E: Hazelnuts, almonds, sunflower seeds.

"Antioxidants are very important substances for the health and well-being of the whole body..."

Additional substances

Apart from antioxidants there is a range of other nutrients that are believed to have specific health benefits to the eye as well as generally. Here are some of these outlined with the foods in which you can find them present.

Vitamin D: Is thought to help reduce the risk of macular degeneration developing. Sunlight can stimulate the skin to produce Vitamin D naturally, so being out in the sun for short periods of time is sufficient to keep your level up.

Foods containing Vitamin D: Orange juice fortified with Vitamin D, salmon, mackerel, sardines, milk.

Zinc: Helps get Vitamin A from certain foods such as carrots so the chemical needed by retinal cells for seeing can be produced, reducing the risk of night blindness. Zinc may also play a role in reducing risk of advanced macular degeneration.

Foods containing Zinc: Beef, oysters, turkey.

Beta-carotene: Can be used by the eye to produce the type of Vitamin A used to make the chemical needed by retinal cells for sight. A lack of this chemical can cause problems seeing at night. Beta-carotene therefore helps protect against night blindness.

Foods containing Beta-carotene: Carrots, sweet potatoes, spinach, butternut squash.

Bioflavonoids (Flavonoids): The body releases antioxidants as it uses up bioflavonoids. The strength of the antioxidants can be stronger than Vitamins C and E. They are thought to protect against cataracts and macular degeneration.

Foods containing Bioflavonoids: tea, red wine, legumes, citrus fruits, bilberries, cherries, blueberries, soy products.

Lutein and Zeaxanthin: Lutein and Zeaxanthin are very similar substances found naturally in the retina. It is thought that good levels of them help to maintain good pigmentation and resistance to free radical forming processes. Good pigmentation of the retina is thought to protect against the effects of UV radiation and macular degeneration in particular.

Foods containing Lutein and Zeaxanthin: Spinach, turnip greens, squash, collard greens, kiwifruit, red peppers, yellow corn.

Omega-3 Fatty Acids: May help prevent dry eyes primarily, due to them being essential for healthy cell membranes and therefore cell integrity.

Foods containing Omega-3 Fatty Acids: Fish such as salmon, mackerel and herring, flaxseed oil and fish oils, ground flaxseeds, walnuts.

Selenium: When combined with Beta-carotene and Vitamins C and E, may reduce risk of advanced AMD.

Foods containing Selenium: Seafood (shrimp, crab, salmon, halibut), Brazil nuts, enriched noodles, brown rice.

It should be said that while these vitamins and substances are essential for a healthy and balanced body, the specific benefits are not agreed or guaranteed by all the research. However, many eye specialists and eye health organisations do recommend these substances to patients suffering a variety of eye conditions. The general feeling in the profession is that making sure your diet incorporates these substances is an important consideration when advising about how to give your eyes the best chance of remaining healthy for longer.

Tips

Supplements are a great way to get the nutrients needed for the eyes, particularly if you are someone with a smaller than average daily food consumption due to low appetite. In the last few years, more eye supplement tablets have come on the market, combining many of the supplements and vitamins mentioned above.

The benefits of these supplement tablets are that you make sure you are getting all the substances in a daily dose when you cannot be sure that your diet or cooking methods are providing you sufficiently with them. It is important to make sure that the dose of supplements is not exceeded, because consuming more doesn't make it better for you and can be unhealthy.

The packaging will have the directions for use labelled for guidance, so read it or get advice as some supplements may not be advised for smokers. Let your optician and doctor know that you are taking the supplements at your next appointment, so they can monitor and advise you accordingly.

#4 KNOW THE SIGNS AND ACT FAST

One of the keys to keeping your vision good is knowing when you need to seek professional help. This is so important because, as with many health conditions, the faster you act the more likely a worst case scenario can be avoided. Over the years I have come across many cases of people who did and didn't act quickly, with a variety of results.

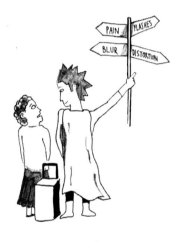

The great memories are ones like Mr Findley, a father in his late 30s, who phoned in with concerns so we arranged for him to come in to see me straight away. He came in reporting a slight blurring in his left eye two days earlier and a strange feeling in the eye when he moved it about fast. The strange thing to me was that Mr Findley had always had poor sight in the left eye and depended almost exclusively on the right eye for all his seeing.

So I was a little surprised that he would notice slight changes in the left eye's sight, unless something more was going on. Having had a thorough look at his eye, it was evident that he had suffered an almost complete detachment of his left retina, meaning that the layer made up of all the cells responsible for seeing had peeled off like wallpaper. Because he hadn't been used to great vision in the left eye anyway, it wasn't too much of a problem for him sight-wise, but I arranged for him to be seen at the local eye hospital straight away for treatment and investigation of the right eye.

Following investigation at the hospital, it turned out that his right eye had also developed two small tears of the retina, for which they treated him. He was told later that he had been at risk of an imminent detachment of the right eye's retina, and it could have happened at any time. The comment really knocked him back, because he realised that it would have meant complete blindness in both eyes – a prospect terrifying at any age, but perhaps more so when you have a young family.

Had Mr Findley thought to himself 'I'll wait a few weeks to see if it gets better since that is my worse eye anyway', his story might have had a very different ending. It's important to develop a relationship with your optical practice that makes you comfortable enough to call in with your concerns, and don't be afraid to come for an earlier eye test appointment should you experience problems.

Some conditions are so urgent that you should by-pass your optician and go directly to eye casualty at the nearest hospital eye department. Here we will look at some of the sudden symptoms that could arise and the action you should take.

Sudden changes to sight

When you notice a significant sudden change in your sight or eye, it usually needs attention by your optician or doctor; it should not be ignored. Here is a selection of relatively common sudden visual changes.

Flashes of light - These are bright, quite distinct and usually appear as an arc in the side of the vision. It is usually seen in dark conditions and is described by the sufferer to be like an electrical spark. These flashes are due to rattling of the transparent sack which holds the vitreous gel in your eyes. The sack is a bit like cling film and is loosely held to the back of the eye. When this 'cling film' sack rattles it creates the flashing lights described.

The flashes are not a problem specifically, but require investigation to make sure there is no tear in the sack which would increase the risk of a detached retina. Seek urgent advice from your optician, and they will advise you based on your circumstance. You may be referred by your optician to the hospital eye department for investigation based on their findings. In my experience, the majority of cases show no sign of damage, so no treatment is needed.

Shadows in your vision - Any awareness of shadowed areas (not just one or two floating particles in the eye), in any part of the vision, requires urgent investigation at a hospital eye department. You could seek advice from your optician over the phone first if it is in working hours but otherwise you should go straight to eye casualty. Any shadows in your sight could be areas where you no longer have sight.

There could be several causes for the loss of sight, but they will require investigation and appropriate treatment where necessary. The longer you leave it, the less likely it can be helped. Migraines may cause temporary shadows or loss of sight, but this usually returns to normal after several minutes to an hour.

Sudden central blur or distortions - Blur or distortion restricted to the central sight is not likely to be due to needing a change of glasses. It is more likely to be due to an issue in the central area of the retina called the macula. This can have several causes so needs urgent investigation to prevent permanent damage to the sight. If you are in any doubt then why not call your optician or GP for advice? These symptoms will most likely need investigation by the hospital eye department.

Shower of dust like floaters - This type of floater is linked with a retinal detachment, the condition in which the retina comes away from the back of the eye, causing sight damage. Typically these floaters come in large numbers, and have been described as being like 'tobacco dust.' Do not confuse them with normal floaters which come in very small numbers. If you are experiencing this, then a direct visit to the nearest eye casualty is advised, particularly if you are also experiencing dark shadows in your sight.

"It's important to remember that many conditions do not have symptoms or they may have such subtle ones that you may quite easily miss them."

Red & painful eyes

Any painful redness of the eyes should be investigated urgently by your optician. It is not unusual to get red eyes from time to time for a variety of reasons, but when it is painful your optician needs to make sure it is not an infection like bacterial conjunctivitis or an inflammatory condition like iritis. These conditions can become very serious to your sight or general health if not treated early. You may be referred on for treatment if necessary.

This is a selection of some of the more common conditions that may come on suddenly. It's important to remember that many conditions do not have symptoms or they may have such subtle ones that you could quite easily miss them. That's why you have regular scheduled sight test appointments, so no matter whether you feel everything is great or not, keep your regular sight test appointment so your optician can check for signs of any problems. The peace of mind you'll feel after being told everything is healthy and well will be worth it.

Family history and risk factors

Another aspect of learning to see the signs and symptoms requiring attention is knowing your family history of eye conditions or any risk factors affecting your family. The benefit of knowing your status means that you can be aware of areas of care you need to take more notice of.

For example, if your mother has glaucoma it doubles your chance of getting glaucoma. If you know this and you inform your optician, you will be monitored more frequently than if your mother didn't have glaucoma. If your father has macular degeneration, you may be advised to look at your nutritional intake, stop smoking and so on. Family history may still affect you even if the family member is deceased so mention it to your optician. It's surprising the number of people who think that family history doesn't count any more when the person in their family dies.

Other risk factors include having a high prescription for glasses (short-sightedness in particular) and ethnicity is the other big one. So for example, many Afro-Caribbeans are not aware that they are more at risk of glaucoma simply because of their ethnicity. There is also a high presence of sickle-cell in the Afro-Caribbean society, a condition affecting the blood and capable of causing burst blood vessels and temporary visual loss in the eye, all of which requires regular monitoring.

Another example is the fact that diabetes has a particularly high presence in the Asian community, requiring regular screening and monitoring on at least an annual basis. Awareness that you are in a higher risk group or that you have a family history of sight problems should motivate you to do better in keeping up regular eye test appointments; it really is for your benefit.

 Tips

If you are having a serious problem and you are not sure what to do, you can call your optician on the telephone and check if they would advise you to go straight to the eye casualty department, your doctor or whether they want you to come in to have an eye test.

#5 IF YOU VALUE YOUR SIGHT, INVEST IN IT

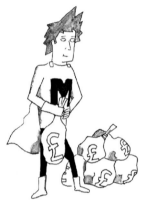

Having worked extensively throughout the country over the last 10 years in nearly every professional situation, a common finding is that everyone everywhere places 'precious' status on their sight, making your sight one of the most valuable commodities you would care to own. So why is it that so many of us actively seek out the cheapest, if not free, sight test available on the market?

I recall a conversation with a woman several years ago about a half-price sight test promotion I was running for my practice. An absolute bargain I thought, given that my business and I took great pride in offering an outstanding service with much attention to the detail of our patients' eye care. Her response was simply, "Why would I pay £12.50 for a sight test when I could go down the road and get one for free?" Yet she was happy to go and have her nails done for £25 every other week at the nail studio across the road.

We all love a bargain when it's on offer, and who can blame anyone for that? It is an instinctive reaction for many and a financially astute one at that. But, when put in the context of looking after your most precious asset, it doesn't sound quite as good an investment after all. The implication here is that there is no difference in quality or service between the opticians that charge £100, £20 and nothing for their eye test.

The most valuable commodity that any optical practice has is the optician's chair time and the presence of a dispensing optician. The optician that tests your eyes is also called an optometrist and has a minimum of four years' training including a degree before they can be registered with the general optical council (GOC). The dispensing optician, often mistaken for an optical assistant, has at least three years' training in all the technical ins and outs of dispensing glasses and lenses, and must also be registered with the GOC in order to work.

As an optometrist, my training covers all aspects of the work of a dispensing optician, but I would never run an optical business without a dispensing optician, due to their speciality in dealing with all the potential complexities of dispensing eyewear products. All optical practices are not the same, just as all supermarkets are not the same. It doesn't necessarily make one better than the other because they may be catering for different sectors of the market.

The cost of glasses and the service you get from your optician should hopefully be based on two things: the quality of the products they are offering and the quality of the professional service. A quality professional service might mean that they invest in one or more dispensing opticians, rather than just in-house trained optical assistants, or they give you more time for your eye test with the optician or they invest in the best technology to give you the best assessment of your eyes' health.

Cost should not be the only basis on which you choose an optician; the overall experience should justify why you are going there. Think of choosing an optician as an investment in your sight; you can get a recommendation from friends or consider some of the following factors.

"All optical practices are not the same, just as all supermarkets are not the same."

What is important?

- Time spent on your eye test - Time should not limit the full range of tests that your optician wants done from taking place. Having enough time allows your optician to answer all your questions and gives them time to elaborate and give proactive advice.

- Rapport and relationship with your optician is important. Having a good relationship with your optician and the staff in the practice is a much underrated part of the experience of having your eyes tested or buying glasses. In my experience, when people have a good relationship with me or my other colleagues, they are quick to let us know of any problems they may be having. They are also more likely to ask all the questions they want, and they tend to have a lasting relationship of care with us.

- What you get for your money. Whatever you pay or don't pay for your eye test, you will be entitled to great care regardless of price, so don't expect anything less. If you are paying budget prices, are you getting budget products and services?

Tips

- If you are worried about the cost of glasses, never feel under pressure to buy your glasses from the same practice where you had your eyes tested. You are entitled to take your prescription away with you and shop around. I do believe that it may be to your advantage to complete your whole care in one place rather than going elsewhere. This is because all your information will be available to your optician throughout the chain of care, and they will presumably know you better too.

When choosing a new optician I would advise that you do some initial research into their prices, products and services. That way you increase the likelihood that all your expectations will be met and a long-lasting relationship can be forged.

- Be honest about the fact that you are on a budget, then it's up to your optician to let you know if they can provide you with the right solution within your budget. If you are still not sure then feel free to take your prescription away and look elsewhere.

AFTERWORD

I hope that having read this book you now have a better understanding of the eye test process, your eyes and what you could be doing to look after them. Having had a great eye test, it is important to make sure that you also get great advice about the right lenses and products for you. This is an area that a qualified dispensing optician is expert in, so don't be afraid to ask them your difficult questions.

Occasionally I come across the patient that is taken aback by how different the eye test experience appears now compared to what they recall of their last eye test, which was invariably many years ago. The biggest change in the eye test in recent years is the introduction of newer and ever-advancing technology into the tests. The future of the eye test continues to be an exciting one that will mean opticians being able to look through to the back of your eyes with unprecedented levels of detail.

Furthermore, we will be able to do so in 3-D and monitor disease changes more accurately from visit to visit, because within seconds these devices can take tens of thousands of scans and produce a host of useful data. While the technology and equipment is already available, I would expect it to become more mainstream in the coming years.

However the future of the eye test and eye care pan out, one thing is for certain, and that is it will continue to advance in many if not all areas. The profession strives to continually improve our ability to care for you, the patient, and help you maintain maximum sight now and in the future through better information, technology and professional advancements.

ABOUT THE AUTHOR

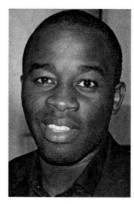

In the last 10 years, Martin Oguzie has gained a wealth of experience working for many of the well known high street opticians and many lesser known smaller independent opticians throughout the country. Martin holds postgraduate qualifications specialising in low vision and ageing, the management of cataract and ocular therapeutics. He has also enjoyed a successful period of practice ownership, an experience that reflects his broad understanding of the eye care industry.

His professional passion is the promotion of eye care awareness and raising the perceived value of the eye test. In a generation where information is so widely available, Martin aims to bring clarity to what is out there. He hopes to make more of us understand our own personal responsibilities in the care of our eyes and, in doing so, the goal is to help reduce the nation's incidence of preventable blindness.

For all the latest updates of what Martin is up to, connect and contact him on:

www.martinoguzie.com

www.twitter.com/MartinOguzie

Also comment about this book on twitter using the *#eyeknowbook* tag.

Lightning Source UK Ltd.
Milton Keynes UK
UKOW030624140112

185368UK00002B/4/P